The
ADOLESCENT
UNIT
Work and Teamwork
in Adolescent Psychiatry

Also by Derek Steinberg

Using Child Psychiatry – The Functions and
Operations of a Specialty

The Clinical Psychiatry of Adolescence

The ADOLESCENT UNIT

Work and Teamwork in Adolescent Psychiatry

Edited by

Derek Steinberg

MB BS MPhil DPM FRCPsych

Consultant Psychiatrist, Adolescent Unit,
Bethlem Royal Hospital & The Maudsley Hospital, London;
Honorary Visiting Reader in Psychiatry and
Human Development, University of Surrey, Guildford

A Wiley Medical Publication

JOHN WILEY & SONS

Chichester · New York · Brisbane · Toronto · Singapore

Library of Congress Cataloging-in-Publication Data:
Main entry under title:

The adolescent unit.

  Includes index.
  1. Adolescent psychiatry.   2. Mental health care
teams.   I. Steinberg, Derek.
RJ503.A325   1985   616.89'022   85-22711
ISBN 0 471 90912 2 (pbk.)

British Library Cataloguing in Publication Data:

Steinberg, Derek
  The Adolescent unit: work and teamwork in
  adolescent psychiatry.
  1. Adolescent psychiatry
  I. Title
  616.89'022   RJ503
  ISBN 0 471 90912 2 Pbk

Phototypeset by Dobbie Typesetting Service, Plymouth, Devon
Printed and bound in Great Britain

Contents

Contributors

Adrian Angold BSc MB BS MRCPsych
Wellcome Research Fellow in Mental Health; formerly Registrar, Bethlem Royal Hospital and the Maudsley Hospital

Derek Bolton MPhil PhD
Lecturer in Psychology, Institute of Psychiatry, University of London; Honorary Principal Clinical Psychologist, Adolescent Unit, Bethlem Royal Hospital and the Maudsley Hospital

Christopher Dare BA MB MRCP FRCPsych DPM
Consultant Psychiatrist, Department of Child and Adolescent Psychiatry, Bethlem Royal Hospital and the Maudsley Hospital

Michael Donnellan RMN Certificate in Child and Adolescent Nursing
Charge Nurse, Adolescent Unit, Bethlem Royal Hospital

John Foskett BA
Anglican Hospital Chaplain, Bethlem Royal Hospital and the Maudsley Hospital

Andrea Gilroy BA ATD
Lecturer in Art Therapy, Goldsmiths' College, University of London

Lynette Hughes BA DipSocAdmin DipApplSocStud
Social Worker, Adolescent Unit, Bethlem Royal Hospital and the Maudsley Hospital, and Southwark Social Services Department.

John Lampen MA DipEd
Formerly Headmaster, Shotton Hall School

Diana Lockie DipCOT SROT
Director of Occupational Therapy Services, Bethlem Royal Hospital and the Maudsley Hospital

Jacqueline Merry DipAD ATC
Art Teacher, Bethlem Royal Hospital School; Adolescent Unit, Bethlem Royal Hospital

Brian Molloy BA Teachers' Cert
DipEd (Malad)

Adviser, Special Educational Needs and Provision, Directorate of Education, London Borough of Bexley; formerly Headteacher, Beech House Adolescent Unit School, St Augustine's Hospital, nr Canterbury, Kent

Deirdre Page CertEd

Music Teacher, Bethlem Royal Hospital School; Adolescent Unit, Bethlem Royal Hospital

William Ll Parry-Jones MA MD
FRCPsych DPM

Consultant Psychiatrist, Highfield Family and Adolescent Unit, Warneford Hospital, Oxford; Clinical Lecturer, University of Oxford; Fellow, Linacre College, Oxford

Derek Steinberg MB BS MPhil
DPM FRCPsych

Consultant Psychiatrist, Adolescent Unit, Bethlem Royal Hospital and the Maudsley Hospital; Honorary Visiting Reader in Psychiatry and Human Development, University of Surrey, Guildford

Eric Taylor MA MB BChir
MRCP MRCpsych

Senior Lecturer in Child and Adolescent Psychiatry, Institute of Psychiatry, University of London; Honorary Consultant Psychiatrist, Bethlem Royal Hospital and the Maudsley Hospital

Diane Waller MA(RCA) ATC
DipPsych

Head of Art Therapy Unit, Goldsmiths' College, University of London

Teresa Wilkinson SRN RMN
RNT DipN DipNEd

Tutor, Post-basic Child and Adolescent Psychiatric Nursing, School of Nursing, Bethlem Royal Hospital and the Maudsley Hospital

Judy F Wilson BA
DipApplSocStud CQSW

Social Worker, Adolescent Unit and Children's Department, Bethlem Royal Hospital and the Maudsley Hospital, and Southwark Social Services Department.

Peter Wilson BA DipApplSocStud
DipChild Psychoanalysis

Director, London Youth Advisory Centre; Consultant Psychotherapist, Peper Harow Therapeutic Community; Principal Child Psychotherapist, Camberwell Child Guidance Clinic; Senior Clinical Tutor in Psychotherapy, Institute of Psychiatry, University of London

Jean Winship

Senior Secretary, Adolescent Unit, Bethlem Royal Hospital and the Maudsley Hospital

Barry Wynn Cert Ed DipArt
Ther RDTh DipPsych

Groupwork Organiser, Family Service Unit, London; Secretary, British Association of Dramatherapists

Preface

In the broad field of adolescent psychiatry there is work, multidisciplinary work, and teamwork. Common usage among professional workers sometimes gives the impression that these terms are more or less equivalent, perhaps even synonymous, an assumption which might follow from the widespread belief that teamwork is a good thing, and that all work, multidisciplinary or otherwise, should properly aspire to it. Moreover, the unspoken argument seems to run: where multidisciplinary teamwork proves problematic for any reason the difficulties that arise must somehow be overcome in the interests of a unified approach.

This is only partly true; I have no doubt that the work of helping adolescents in trouble, researching their difficulties and educating the people involved requires the collaboration of people with many different kinds of skill and experience. To this extent it is an assumption throughout this book that multidisciplinary work in this field is not merely desirable or advisable but is a necessity; what is not so clear, and is certainly not assumed in this book, is that whatever the task the best way of cooperating is as a team.

What, after all, is a 'team'? Sometimes it is no more than a convenient collective label for a group of people working together, whatever their professions, and is used where for various reasons such terms as group, band, troupe or squad might be considered inappropriate. But no such label is without some significance (in which context the teaching hospital tradition of using the word 'firm', complete with chiefs, is of interest). Later in the book it is suggested that the word team conveys the idea of unity in a common purpose, with individuality and individual action being subordinated to the beliefs and methods of the team, either by consensus or by acceptance of the authority of the team's leader. This is necessary for some aspects of work but by no means for all, and the drift towards 'teamwork', for all its advantages, needs to be countered by a reminder of what individual people contribute to multiprofessional work, and of what may be lost when the concept of teamwork is given automatic priority. The beneficent team can then become a tyrant, with the innovation and flair of individuals, the needs of a particular adolescent's case or the wishes of patients and families being subjugated to the way of thinking of 'the team'. The point is not to dismiss the value of teamwork, but to remember that it involves losses as well as gains, and that whether one is planning for an elaborate service, a specific project or a particular piece of work with an adolescent the advantages of individuality need to be set firmly against the advantages of a tight 'team philosophy'.

The authors of the chapters in this book were asked to contribute because they work in their own way and seem able to work successfully with others who do the same, something which, incidentally, I think is an important capacity for adults to demonstrate to adolescents. In their chapters they describe what they actually do, which I hope will be the main interest and value of the book. They discuss their work in relation to others, but the emphasis is on what they do themselves, how they see their work and how they spend their day rather than on a detailed account of the vicissitudes of collaboration.

Most of the contributors work, or have worked, in the Adolescent Unit at Bethlem Royal Hospital, or like Diane Waller and Andrea Gilroy are closely associated with us through training programmes. Three are friends from outside rather than immediate colleagues: John Lampen, William Parry-Jones and Brian Molloy, the latter in the special position of having worked for several years at the Unit School at Bethlem before going on to Beech House Adolescent Unit at Canterbury. I am enormously grateful to them all, particularly to those not naturally disposed to get into print, and who found the task one they would have preferred to avoid.

I want to thank also Patrick West, Patricia Sharp and Verity Waite of John Wiley and Sons Ltd for their assistance at every stage, my wife Gill for compiling the indexes, and my daughters Kate and Anna for helping in the recurring task of collating an astonishing amount of paper.

Derek Steinberg
Bethlem Royal Hospital
January 1986

1 Social Work on the Bridge

Lynette Hughes & Judy Wilson

On this bridge of our professional development (Fig. 1.1) we illustrate how, despite the differences in our histories, we have discovered many shared influences and common themes in our backgrounds. Since first meeting in 1977, as social workers on the Adolescent Unit at the Bethlem Royal and Maudsley Hospitals, we have developed together many professional interests that have united us on the bridge that spans the space between our histories.

———◆———

In looking at 'Social Work on the Bridge', we wish to use the metaphor of a bridge rather differently from the way we have used it in our introductory illustration. The bridge that links a psychiatric inpatient unit to the world outside is the place where the expectations, needs and priorities of the unit, its staff and its patients meet those of the professional agencies and the families from without. It is the place both where firm and creative alliances are made and where severe conflicts are fought out. Whatever the exact nature of the interaction, it inevitably contains within it seeds of tension. The temptation is strong at this point to develop the metaphor of the bridge into images involving Simon and Garfunkel's 'Troubled Waters', Horatio's 'Holding the Bridge', the never-ending task of painting the Forth Bridge, or the suicides off Clifton Bridge; but we shall restrain ourselves!

The following three case examples typify some of the tensions that exist on this bridge between an in-patient adolescent unit and the outside.

Everyone was delighted with the way in which 14-year-old Lorraine had blossomed in the Adolescent Unit and begun to enjoy life after being withdrawn and psychotic on admission. When a ward disco was arranged there was disagreement between those staff who assumed she should attend and those who emphasised the need to act on the wishes of her strict Seventh Day Adventist parents, known to be opposed to dancing.

Fifteen-year-old Martin's parents had separated one year before his admission to the psychiatric unit, and his mother, with whom he lived, had legal custody. His father had been awarded reasonable access. Both parents visited him regularly in the unit, but his weekends were spent at home with his mother. One weekend, when Martin's mother was away for a few days and Martin was the only adolescent left on the unit over the weekend, his father asked if Martin could stay with him overnight. As Martin's mother had not

1

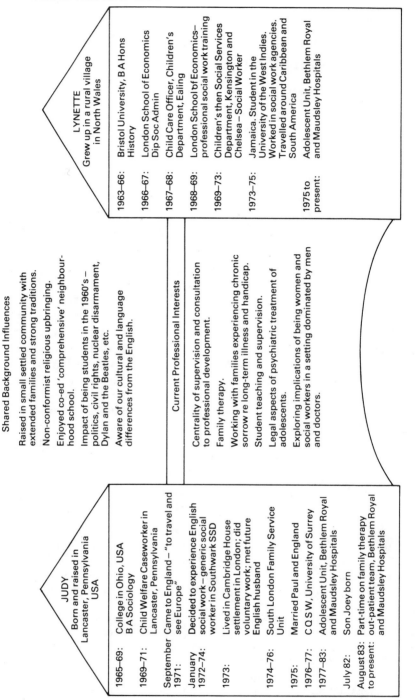

JUDY
Born and raised in
Lancaster, Pennsylvania
USA

1965–69: College in Ohio, USA
          B A Sociology

1969–71: Child Welfare Caseworker in
          Lancaster, Pennsylvania

September Came to England – "to travel and
1971:   see Europe"

January   Decided to experience English
1972–74: social work – generic social
          worker in Southwark SSD

1973:   Lived in Cambridge House
          settlement in London; did
          voluntary work; met future
          English husband

1974–76: South London Family Service
          Unit

1975:   Married Paul and England

1976–77: C Q S W, University of Surrey

1977–83: Adolescent Unit, Bethlem Royal
          and Maudsley Hospitals

July 82: Son Joey born

August 83: Part-time on family therapy
to present: out-patient team, Bethlem Royal
          and Maudsley Hospitals

Shared Background Influences

Raised in small settled community with
extended families and strong traditions.

Non-conformist religious upbringing.

Enjoyed co-ed 'comprehensive' neighbour-
hood school.

Impact of being students in the 1960's –
politics, civil rights, nuclear disarmament,
Dylan and the Beatles, etc.

Aware of our cultural and language
differences from the English.

Current Professional Interests

Centrality of supervision and consultation
to professional development.

Family therapy.

Working with families experiencing chronic
sorrow re long-term illness and handicap.

Student teaching and supervision.

Legal aspects of psychiatric treatment of
adolescents.

Exploring implications of being women and
social workers in a setting dominated by men
and doctors.

LYNETTE
Grew up in a rural village
in North Wales

1963–66: Bristol University, B A Hons
          History

1966–67: London School of Economics
          Dip Soc Admin

1967–68: Child Care Officer, Children's
          Department, Ealing

1968–69: London School of Economics—
          professional social work training

1969–73: Children's then Social Services
          Department, Kensington and
          Chelsea – Social Worker

1973–75: Jamaica. Student in the
          University of the West Indies.
          Worked in social work agencies.
          Travelled around Caribbean and
          South America

1975 to   Adolescent Unit, Bethlem Royal
present: and Maudsley Hospitals

Fig. 1.1   The bridge of our professional development

consented to such an overnight stay, the unit staff felt they had to refuse. Martin and his father were very angry.

The area team social worker was extremely concerned about the deteriorating physical condition of 13-year-old Jane and the effect of her obsessional rituals on her family. He requested urgent admission to the Adolescent Unit, as did Jane's parents. Jane had initially been referred to the Unit for admission by a consultant in another psychiatric hospital where Jane had had two previous admissions, and where, following crisis admissions requested by her parents, she had twice been prematurely discharged by them. In view of this history of ambivalent parental authority and of their own recent assessment of the family, the Adolescent Unit had decided that Jane could be treated successfully as an inpatient only if the local authority applied either to the Juvenile Court for a care order or to make Jane a ward of court. The area team social worker was concerned that in his department the machinery for preparing legal proceedings in such a situation was too protracted to meet the urgent needs of the case, and he was also hesitant about the appropriateness of using child care legislation where there were psychiatric problems.

These three examples together illustrate how the bridge is the meeting place of different cultural and religious values, of different ideas of what is most therapeutic for the adolescent, of different theoretical frameworks in assessing and handling a psychiatric crisis and of the differing sources of authority in decision making – parental, clinical, personal and child care or mental health legislation. Among the professionals in the multidisciplinary team in an adolescent inpatient unit, it is most often the social worker who occupies the central point on the bridge between the inside and outside and who works to facilitate and inform communication between the two. It is this aspect of the social worker's role that we wish to discuss.

A great deal has been written about the aims and tasks of social work with adolescents generally (eg. Laycock 1970), about the role of social work in child psychiatry (eg. Lask 1981) and about the difficulty in distinguishing between distinctive professional roles and individual skills, personality, and experience when looking at the contribution of one profession within a multidisciplinary team (Rowbottom 1978). We are conscious of drawing on ideas developed in this broad background, but in this chapter we shall be focusing more narrowly. We shall not be attempting to offer a blueprint for the role of social workers on adolescent inpatient units; we know of social workers on other units who interpret their roles very differently, and we are aware that the role we have developed is related to the nature of the unit in which we work. Nor shall we attempt to describe all aspects of our work, for example as family and individual therapists, student supervisors, conveners of parents' groups or consultants to members of other disciplines, but will focus on the social worker's role on the bridge between the inpatient unit and the outside.

On The Bridge – With Colleagues and Alone

What are the tasks of those who work on this bridge?

1 Representing the inside to the outside

(a) Discussing assessment and admission policies with referrers.
(b) Communicating details of an adolescent's progress to his family or outside social worker.
(c) Making clear to the family how their participation in treatment can help the adolescent.
(d) Applying to other agencies for suitable resources and help for the adolescents.

2 Representing the outside to the inside

(a) Reminding the 'inside' team of the constant need to communicate appropriately with those outside. For example, giving an outside social worker sufficient notice of a ward round discussion; informing the closely-involved parents of a 16-year-old of the decision to prescribe medication even where the adolescent is able and willing to give his consent.
(b) Maintaining the perspective of an inpatient's previous history and life outside the unit, to illuminate events within the unit, eg. looking at how staff reactions around an adolescent may mirror his family dynamics; checking progress in previous residential placements the better to understand current progress and failures. Maintaining this perspective can be difficult for those involved in daily struggles with an adolescent.
(c) Providing the 'inside' with general knowledge and information from the outside, eg. child care legislation; availability of resources.

3 Facilitating direct communication between inside and outside

(a) Defining liaison work with outside agencies as being equally important to direct clinical work.
(b) Encouraging a wide range of staff to spend some time on the bridge and providing supervision for those wishing for the first time to undertake regular work there, eg. a charge nurse's supervision of a staff nurse's consultative role with a children's home.
(c) Formalising regular, shared planning meetings between members of each discipline, the adolescent and his family.

  This list could clearly be extended. Of course, it covers tasks undertaken by members of all disciplines. In standing on this bridge, we acknowledge that, as social workers, we are, in fact, usually surrounded by colleagues of other disciplines, also firmly committed to working with the families of inpatients, to liaising or consulting with outside professionals and to exploring the normality of an adolescent's life outside the hospital. However, even when thus happily surrounded, there are factors that can give social workers a particular position on the bridge, namely their employment by an outside authority, the local authority Social Services Department;

their statutory powers under child care and mental health legislation; their knowledge of local authority and voluntary societies' resources for adolescents; and their training in considering the legal, financial, cultural, religious, political and social aspects of client functioning. Often the social worker will also have more experience of interviewing families, but this will clearly vary, depending on the experience of other team members.

While some tension always exists on the bridge between community and unit expectations and needs, standing on it, surrounded by like-minded colleagues, can be a relatively comfortable position. Finding ourselves as social workers suddenly alone on the bridge can therefore be disconcerting. At times of crisis, the differences between disciplines tend to become more clearly defined, and the line between professional collaboration and professional isolation can be very fine. Nurses, teachers, occupational therapists and, to a lesser extent, psychiatrists, then understandably give priority to their responsibility for the immediate care of the adolescent inpatient group, and become more inward looking. The social worker remains freer to choose to look outward from the unit as well as inwards, and to continue to emphasise external considerations as still being essential to any decision making, a freedom that colleagues of other disciplines may see as representing too much commitment to external factors.

At times of crisis, too, differences of philosophy and theoretical orientation become highlighted, and the team that usually succeeds in combining a range of differing models within its therapeutic repertoire has, in crisis, to face more clearly the conflicts between the models, eg. medical 'sickness' model versus family systems model. While often frustrating and uncomfortable, such theoretical differences are in our view also inevitable and exciting (Lampen 1981). We feel strongly that a team that does not have the courage to face its theoretical differences directly not only misses the opportunity of using fully the range of available skills but also runs the risk of confusing its clients by the overt or covert differences of approach by team members. Of course, facing differences can be paralysing if it does not lead on to clear decision making about which course to follow amid the ambiguities and competing requirements of different treatment approaches (Eisenberg 1975), and in our opinion the role of the medical consultant as an effective decision maker in such situations is crucial. Our commitment to exploring our theoretical differences within the multidisciplinary team does not, however, diminish the discomfort of finding that, in such crises, our views can place us, as social workers, firmly alone on the bridge.

Our image of social work on the bridge sounds like an amalgam of the two old clichés – that of the traditional hospital social worker's role as being concerned only with 'where the patient came from and where the patient went', with no involvement in between; and that of the field social worker as representing the family to institutions, and *vice versa*. There are many ways in which the role we are describing challenges these clichés, not least the clinical treatment input of the social worker and the importance of being a firm member of the 'residential' team, not just a visitor from outside. The clichés are, however, a significant reminder of the importance in many settings of the social work role of standing on the bridge between the inside and the outside.

We see this position as one of striving to maintain a dynamic balance between the differing requirements and expectations of inside and out; the point of balance will vary with the circumstances of each situation, and we will not always agree with colleagues about the placing of this point. Our argument is that, in a psychiatric unit for adolescents, whatever the disagreements about the right point of balance, the bridge will have a distinctive and particular significance which we would relate to two closely-linked factors, (a) the concept of authority as a central factor is working with adolescents, and (b) the complexity of the legal framework.

Authority and The Legal Framework

The concept of authority

The centrality of the concept of authority in working with disturbed adolescents has been fully developed by a number of authors (Winnicott, 1971; Bruggen, 1975). They have written about the need for adolescents to come into contact with adults who are unafraid to use their authority consistently, clearly, in a non-retaliatory manner, and if necessary unpopularly, in order that the adolescents may in their turn develop a confidence in their own autonomy and develop their own authority. Adult authority is most clearly seen by adolescents in decision making and in the implementation of rules that provide structure and standards.

A central task in the treatment of adolescents, even where a medical model may be used to define their problems as sickness, is thus defining and making explicit who, at any one time, has the authority for making which decision about what. Authority springs from many sources. A doctor, for example, has a professional authority that arises from technical expertise, while medicine as a profession, unlike social work, carries also a traditional authority arising from its long history. Social workers, however, have a statutory authority under child care and mental health legislation. Cultural and religious traditions and practice provide an authority that informs much decision making, while the second case example, that of Martin and his divorced parents, illustrates authority arising both from the law and from personal attributes and personality. Making a clear point of differentiating between the various sources of authority can be an active therapeutic intervention. For example, an anorexic adolescent of under sixteen, with a dangerously low weight, may be admitted to hospital on the agreement of her parents but by dint of the consultant using the full weight of his medical authority to influence the parents' decision, and by expressing his willingness to invoke mental health legislation if necessary. When the adolescent reaches a safe weight, even though the psychiatric team may prefer her to remain longer in hospital while family issues begin to be worked with, the parents may be told clearly that discharge is now totally dependent on their decision about when they feel confident to begin to look after their child again.

Authority derived from professional, cultural, religious, traditional or personal sources can never, however, be appropriate if it is in contradiction to the relevant legal authority. With adolescents under sixteen the legal authority for most major decision making lies outside the unit, with the parents or area team social workers, and the unit social worker's task of reminding busy staff of this reality can be as crucial as that of drawing parents' and psychiatrists' attention to the increasing civil and legal rights of an adolescent who is opposed to their advice. The social worker is in a strong position *vis-à-vis* most other staff to take on this role of 'clarifying the source of authority'. Firstly, by nature of being less directly involved in the day-to-day care of the adolescents, the social worker is under less pressure to be drawn into competing with the natural parents for the role of 'best parent'; and by being more distant from the adolescents' anger at their parents' shortcomings, is in an easier position to appreciate that these parents, whatever their shortcomings, will be the only family the adolescents have long after the unit's staff have forgotten their names. The first case example at the beginning of this chapter, about the daughter of strict, Seventh Day Adventist parents, presents an instance that gives rise to such tensions.

The second factor which puts the social worker in a strong position to clarify the source of authority is her knowledge of the relevant legislation.

The legal framework

Bruggen (1975) speaks of the law as being, like a rule, 'a convenient yardstick' over which issues of authority and autonomy can be worked out. Probably no client group has the possibility of being affected by such a wide range of legislation as are

Table 1.1 Legislation affecting adolescents.

Child care law, eg. reception into care Juvenile criminal law Matrimonial law Law relating to all adolescents, eg. age of buying alcohol		Mental health legislation
Adolescents in children's homes	Adolescents in psychiatric units	Adults in psychiatric wards
Law relating to all adults of 16 years plus, eg. DHSS benefit entitlement; consent to treatment		
Civil rights		

adolescents in a psychiatric unit. Table 1.1, which compares them with children in residential care and with adult psychiatric patients, illustrates the complexity.

The law that relates generally to all adolescents is well-known for its contradictions and ambiguities, reflecting the nature of adolescence as between childhood and adulthood (Rae 1982). The regular, public debate over the issues of the age of girls' consent to sexual intercourse and the allied questions of consent to contraception and termination, as well as over consent to medical treatment in general, is a clear example of this (Gaylin 1982). Not surprisingly, therefore, a setting that brings together the range of different legal frameworks outlined above offers scope for considerable confusion and conflict, eg. the possible conflict between the authority of a care order to maintain a 16-year-old in a residential setting, which may be a hospital, against his will; and the right of a 16-year-old to consent to medical treatment and more specifically to psychiatric hospital admission (Child Care Act 1980; Family Law Reform Act 1969; Mental Health Act 1983).

Case illustrations

Two examples may help to illustrate the close relationship between the therapeutic management of adolescents and the legal definition of authority, rights and responsibilities.

Fifteen-year-old Paul's family consisted of an older sister of twenty and his mother. Since his admission it had become clear that it was his sister who, because of her personality and capabilities, exercised most of the maternal and adult authority in the household. In negotiating arrangements for Paul to spend weekends at home, it was easy to forget that it was only Paul's mother who had the legal authority to consent to arrangements, and the social worker sometimes needed to remind colleagues that acting on this reality was both legally and therapeutically necessary.

John was recovering well from his depressive breakdown when his sixteenth birthday approached. Despite his constant statements about wanting to discharge himself, it was clear that he had responded well to his parents' new-found capacity to withstand his demands, and he had made no attempt to run away or refuse medication as they had unitedly and firmly told him they wished him to accept treatment. John knew that when he was sixteen he had the right to decide himself whether or not to accept treatment. As his birthday approached, he became increasingly miserable and two days before his birthday he took an overdose. The psychiatrist who saw him at the time was seriously concerned about his mood, recognised fully its relation to his birthday, and decided that he was prepared to recommend that John be compulsorily detained under the Mental Health Act. This decision provided John with considerable relief, despite his protestations to the contrary. By the following day, when the social worker saw him, he was much more relaxed, and his certainty now that the only alternative to remaining voluntarily was compulsory detention had freed him to be able to decide that he wished to be an informal patient. The social worker felt unable to agree to the application for compulsory detention, although she made it clear to the parents that they still had the option of making the application themselves.

This second case illustrates not only the changing legal powers of parents and adolescents and the possible clinical impact on adolescents of any change in their legal status, but also highlights the different roles of doctor and social worker when acting under the authority of mental health legislation and the scope for differences in interpretation of legal requirements. Some may view such a disagreement between doctor and social worker as a sign of the collapse of the therapeutic authority of the psychiatric team. It certainly has that potential. We would argue, however, that, if handled openly and well within the multidisciplinary team, with doctor and social worker seen by their clients to be in close and thoughtful discussion on the issues, such disagreement may even serve to enhance the therapeutic authority of the team.

Older adolescents' acquisition of legal and personal authority is a gradual, ambiguous and variable process. Professionals who are able to clarify the extent and limits of their authority over their adolescent patients and avoid the temptation of easy solutions, while remaining clear themselves about what course of action will be pursued amid the differences, are then in a position to help their patients in their struggle with their own authority.

Admission and Discharge

Admission and discharge are naturally the times when the bridge is at its busiest and when many of the issues already discussed can be seen both at their clearest and at their most confusing. The writings of Bruggen (1973) on the therapeutic use of clarifying the authority of admission to Hill End Adolescent Unit has had considerable influence on our colleagues and ourselves, but other considerations also have to be taken into account when considering admission to an eclectic hospital unit that uses a number of different therapeutic approaches. Discharge is a topic only sparsely covered in the literature, though Brearley (1982) draws usefully on experience and thinking from a number of different settings. None of the literature with which we are familiar, however, looks at the differing roles and priorities of different disciplines during admission and discharge. The following case examples contrast the social worker's role at such times with the roles of other team members.

A case for urgent admission?

Once a week a referral meeting is held at which representatives from the multidisciplinary team discuss all new referrals. The following referral letter requesting urgent admission was received.

Referral Letter from Child Guidance Clinic Consultant to the Adolescent Unit Consultant

Could you please urgently admit Liza P, an intelligent 15½-year-old girl who has been school refusing for the past one-and-a-half years. She previously enjoyed school and was always top of her class. She is currently very depressed, having become increasingly withdrawn and uncommunicative in the past six months. She rarely leaves her bedroom now except for necessities, refuses to join in family meals, and is eating very little. Having previously been father's pet, she now refuses to speak to him or even to be in the same room. Despite a lot of effort no one seems able to reach her, though her mother probably relates to her best. She has told her mother she no longer wants to go on living, and her mother suspects some of her own sleeping tablets have gone missing.

Liza and her mother have been seen individually by myself and the clinic social worker for the past three months. Her father, Mr P, a prominent barrister, has been seen only once because of pressures of his work, and in fact, since the meeting when Mr P attended, Liza has refused to speak to me at all.

There are two siblings: Joan – 19 years old, no problems and away at college; Henry – 13 years old, on a Supervision Order to the local authority for minor delinquency problems and truancy.

Could you please admit Liza urgently? Mrs P 'can't cope any longer' and is desperate for her daughter to be taken into hospital, though Liza is adamantly against admission and threatens to run away if admitted.

This letter was followed by three phone calls, one each to the Unit's consultant, social worker and head teacher, from their respective counterparts in the community. The doctor reported that Liza had now made superficial cuts to her wrists and was eating less. The child guidance clinic social worker revealed that Mrs P hinted at marital problems, and said her husband told her it was up to her if she wanted to put their daughter 'in a bin'. The social worker went on to say that a lot of effort had gone into trying to involve Mr P, all to no avail, and she hoped his lack of cooperation would not delay admission because Mrs P was at her 'wits end'. Liza's old school counsellor rang to say she had been seeing Liza for just over a year and had just learned that the child guidance clinic were involved and that the Unit was now considering admission. She wanted to convey her extreme concern for this child and hoped the Unit would admit her urgently as Liza had shared some confidential

Table 1.2   Primary considerations and priority rating by main unit disciplines.

Considerations	Social worker	Doctors	Nurses	Teachers
Who is in charge of the child?	●●●	●	●	
Health and mental state	●	●●●	●●●	●
Family and social history	●●●	●●	●	●
Legal issues and children's rights	●●●	●	●	●
Professional network	●●●	●●	●	●●
Adolescent unit needs	●	●●●	●●●	●●
Community resources	●●●	●		●
Informal and unspoken considerations	●	●	●	●
Therapeutic intervention	●●	●●	●●	●●

●●●   Key issue for discipline
●●   Medium priority issue for discipline
●   Lower priority issue for discipline

information about Mr and Mrs P with her. She did not want Liza to know she had telephoned.

In the subsequent discussion each professional discipline tended to give more priority to some areas than others when trying to decide on the most appropriate plan of action. These differing priorities are illustrated in Table 1.2.

Each discipline respected the validity of all these considerations but at times of crisis (such as a request for urgent admission) conflicts frequently arise and making decisions becomes more difficult. We shall discuss each consideration in more detail, to give some idea of the complexities of decision making in a multidisciplinary team, with particular emphasis on the social work role in this process.

Who is in charge?

When discussing any new referral one of the first considerations is who has charge of this child or who has authority to make decisions about her (Bruggen & O'Brian 1984). In this case both Mr and Mrs P have equal legal responsibility. Although each parent can legally give consent to admission in the absence of the other (Guardianship Act 1973), admitting Liza on the authority of only one parent without the agreement of the other would be a precarious start to treatment. Here it appears as if Mrs P is in favour of admission and Mr P is not: if we agreed to admit on Mrs P's request, Mr P could legally discharge Liza within hours if he wished to do so.

Health and mental state

Both the doctors and the nurses are equally concerned about Liza's continuing physical and mental deterioration, despite her outpatient treatment in the local clinic. Her lack of eating and suicidal talk suggest an urgency to her current condition which they believe would be helped by admission before she becomes too entrenched, due to the severity of her symptoms.

Family and social history

From the referral we are able to elicit several important historical details about Liza and her family:

(a) both Liza and Henry are refusing school,
(b) Mrs P is on sleeping tablets,
(c) there are allegedly marital problems between Mr and Mrs P, and
(d) Mr P is reluctant to be involved despite previously having had a very close relationship with his daughter.

To the social worker, in particular, these are all indicators of difficulties within the family, not just with Liza herself, and would prompt the social worker to advocate seeking the family's complete involvement and cooperation before agreeing to admission. On the positive side, Liza's previous school record was very good and the Unit teachers think a quick admission would enable Liza to attend the more protective environment of the Unit school, therefore not jeopardizing the one area of her life that has been successful.

Legal issues and children's rights

In Liza's case there are several areas which are worth considering. For example, when Liza soon becomes 16 years old she will be able legally to discharge herself against parental or medical advice unless she were sectionable under the 1983 Mental Health Act.

On the other hand, could she be made a subject of a care order because of her failure to attend school? In Liza's situation a care order is unlikely to be welcomed by the Social Services Department because of her age, and there are no educational grounds while she has home tuition, as this complies with the Education Department's requirements.

As social workers we feel it is preferable to use normal parental authority, or child care legislation which deals with the general ordinary needs of all children, rather than involve mental health legislation, as long as the adolescent's needs and rights are sufficiently protected.

Professional network

Who else is involved with Liza, and what are their plans? In our experience it is important to establish who is clearly involved professionally with the referred patient so as not to duplicate or undermine their work. For instance, in Liza's case it would be important to find out the degree of Education Welfare's role in view of her long-term non-school attendance. Also what is the school counsellor's role and should she remain involved if Liza were to be admitted? In addition, the Social Services are already involved with Henry, and we would want to know if they were also concerned with Liza. In referrals that already have a number of professionals closely involved there are strong arguments that any new agency should arrange a consultation meeting with all those already involved before deciding whether to make direct contact with the family.

Reder & Kraemer (1980) describe how at the point of referral the dynamics of professional networks may mirror those of the family. They highlight how in order to prevent repeating this process the agency receiving the referral should undertake work with the referring agencies before meeting the family. In Liza's case the professional network seems to be mirroring the family not only by its secret communication but also by the women being over-involved and the men remaining on the periphery. Bruggen & O'Brian (1984) show how a consultation meeting may actually prevent the need for admission to an adolescent unit, while Burck (1978) indicates that families are more likely to take up an offer of new help if there is a clear understanding between the agencies making and receiving the referral.

Adolescent unit needs

At any given time the needs of the adolescent unit itself change and must be taken into consideration. Liza, although very ill physically, is seen by the nurses and teachers as a bright school-refuser and a welcome change from the recent intake of psychotic children. On the other hand, she is also a potential suicide risk and the nurses are worried about their ability to keep a constant watch on her as they are currently short-staffed. However, it is also important to fill vacant beds because both the nursing and teaching levels are assessed on bed occupancy.

Community resources
In considering what is in Liza's best interests, we would want to explore alternatives to hospital admission and whether any local resource would be more appropriate or useful. Although being received into care to a local authority children's home is one such alternative, most homes or day units would be reluctant to admit Liza because of her suicidal threats.

Informal and unspoken considerations
These unspoken considerations can range from the broad quasipolitical issues to more personal concerns. For example, on the political level the Unit may be particularly concerned to demonstrate its value to the community not only because of its local commitment but also in light of the impending Health and Social Services spending cuts. A more personal concern for the doctors is that they would be seen to carry responsibility if she chose to kill herself. In this situation, there is also a collective, largely-unspoken memory of the recent suicide of an outpatient which worries every team member when they hear of Liza's suicidal threats.

Therapeutic interventions
How do all these considerations affect our choice of therapeutic interventions? Everyone agrees about the seriousness of Liza's predicament and her need for urgent help. However, is an assessment for urgent admission the most appropriate way to respond?

Doctors and nurses all feel the need for an urgent assessment for admission because of her rapid deterioration and that, almost certainly, immediate admission will be indicated. They also agree, despite the shortage of nursing staff, that hospital will be a safer place for Liza at present. The teachers, as stated before, also agree that admission as soon as possible is preferable.

The social worker accepts the doctor's preliminary assessment that Liza will probably need admission but strongly asserts that admission should not be arranged without Mr and Mrs P's joint involvement even though, legally, Liza could be admitted with the consent of one parent. The social worker feels the crisis should be used to try to involve Mr P because of his uninvolvement in the past and what she sees as the consequent failure of outpatient treatment. The social worker's firm belief is that Liza's disturbance has a function for this family and that her long-term safety can best be insured by mobilising the resources of the family from the outset. The social worker also feels that a pre-assessment network meeting is necessary in view of all the people involved. She is concerned that a rushed admission could be sabotaged by the parents or others in the network unless they are included at the beginning, and this stands her apart from her medical colleagues who give greater weight at this point to removing Liza speedily to a safe place.

THE OUTCOME

The decision at the referral meeting was that the whole family should be invited for an urgent assessment for admission, but if Liza's father did not attend, and she needed admission, she could still be admitted as soon as possible. A preliminary network meeting was seen as causing too much delay, but all the professionals involved were invited to a discussion following the assessment.

The appointment was held within days; Mr P was unable to come. Mrs P came with Liza, Henry and Joan, and the child guidance clinic social worker. While at the Unit Liza returned from the lavatory, staggering, with an empty pill bottle in her hand. She was admitted immediately with Mrs P's consent. That night she ran off and was reported missing, as she did not return home. The police picked her up the following night, put her on a Place of Safety Order and returned her to the Adolescent Unit. Mr and Mrs P went to the Unit the next morning to visit Liza and to discuss events with the staff. Due to the Place of Safety Order, a case conference of all the professionals involved was arranged for the following week. Liza meanwhile remained very tearful and refused to come out of her room.

CONCLUSION

The complexities of a situation such as Liza's are all too familiar to workers in an adolescent unit. We are equally familiar in a multidisciplinary team with different team members having different viewpoints. Because of this, it is our belief that some discussion between team members is essential, with a view to airing the differences, despite the danger of seeming to be competitive. It is important, as in Liza's case, to look at the possible alternatives and then make a decision so that when the team acts it acts with authority and the differences do not serve to undermine the final decision.

As social workers in an inpatient unit we recognise that it is the consultant who has the final say on whether a patient is in need of admission. But in relation to the various considerations with which a social worker is more familiar due to her experience, we feel it is her duty to make strong representations to the team accordingly, as in Liza's case.

No doubt the social worker would say that had the Unit insisted on Mr P's attendance before the admission, Liza would not have had to increase the level of anxiety even further by running away and involving the police and the Courts, which in turn ensured Mr P's attendance at the Unit. On the other hand, had she not been admitted because of Mr P's non-involvement, she may very well have actually succeeded in committing suicide in a final desperate attempt to secure his attention.

Discharge – case illustration

Alan, who was 15 years old and in care under Section 1, Child Care Act 1980 (voluntary care), had been admitted eight months previously to the Adolescent Unit because of concern about his depression. Soon after his admission, though depressive features remained, staff had to concern themselves more with his aggressive behaviour and limit-testing. Most staff now wished to discharge him quickly because of his persistent disruptive behaviour, which upset the more vulnerable patients, and because of his regular physical attacks on staff at a time of severe nursing understaffing. Alan had already received many warnings that he would be discharged if his behaviour persisted. The social worker's role on the bridge is illustrated in Table 1.3. Although some of the views attributed to the social worker were shared by colleagues, the social worker was the only staff member to raise them all.

One aspect of communication left out of this diagram is the work in staff groups, (see Chapter 17 and 21) which are essential in dealing with the feelings raised by communications such as these!

Conclusions

No discussion of the role of the social worker in a multidisciplinary team can avoid some direct reference to issues of dual accountability: professional and bureaucratic accountability to the Social Services Department outside the hospital, and professional accountability to colleagues of all disciplines and to clients within the hospital. Social workers thus stand on their own professional bridge between two organisations that may sometimes disagree strongly in their views of professional roles, responsibilities and priorities. Within the multidisciplinary team, social workers are often seen as senior and experienced members of staff; within the Social Services Department their experience may be recognised but within the local authority hierarchy their position is near the bottom of the ladder. The current career structure for social workers contributes greatly to this discrepancy for many social workers in child and adolescent psychiatry. Social workers wishing to specialise in aspects of direct client work often move into hospital or clinic settings because of the shortage of opportunities for such specialism within area offices, where the only route for development may be into management. For the same reason, social workers often remain for a long time in the same posts within their multidisciplinary teams, where their continuity and permanence contribute greatly to their influence. Social workers' commitment to working in multidisciplinary teams may lead some Social Services Departments to wonder whether they are only the handmaidens of the consultant, and some multidisciplinary colleagues to wish to forget the social workers' commitment to issues within their employing authority (such as during the recent struggles over the conditions of work of residential social workers). In our experience, however, social workers in such positions are fully aware, on the one hand, of the

Table 1.3 Communications.

From Unit Social Worker to rest of Adolescent Unit Team

- Reminded how rapid discharge replicated Alan's family experiences.
- Urged discussion of how to communicate decision, and how to ease transfer.
- Reminded that discharge, however appropriate, broke Unit's pledge to prepare Alan for hostel placement.
- Argued for some delay in actual discharge to aid preparation.
- Pointed out difficulty outside social worker had in finding any placement quickly for adolescent.
- Informed that local authority's current financial policy prevented all funding of placements outside borough, hence could not use good placement known to Unit.
- Explained that Alan's parents legally able to take him home, despite psychiatric recommendation to contrary.

From Adolescent Unit Social Worker to Family and Outside Social Worker

- Social worker in multidisciplinary team that conveyed decision, but undertook further meetings alone. In these defended Unit's decision, despite own misgivings, and confirmed Unit's deadline.

From Rest of Adolescent Unit Team to Unit Social Worker

- Pointed out staff shortages, seriousness of attacks, previous warnings, welfare of patient group, and stressed that social worker not under direct pressure from these.
- Stated reality that hospital not legally responsible for Alan.
- Agreed that multidisciplinary group would communicate decision to family, but special nurse unable to do follow-up work because of staff shortages.

Between Adolescent Unit Social Worker and Family and Outside Social Worker

- Meetings of all to work with anger and sadness of family (including Alan) over discharge.
- Meetings continued after discharge to break pattern, as family had manoeuvred abrupt angry endings with all previous agencies.
- Social workers pooled information re placements and Unit social worker tried to convey understanding of dilemmas of finding rapid placement, while outside social worker acknowledged Unit's difficulty.
- Unit social worker arranged to be available to outside social worker for consultation over case in future.

ADOLESCENT UNIT

UNIT

WORKER

FAMILY AND OUTSIDE SOCIAL WORKER

UNIT SOCIAL WORKER

extent as well as the limit of their influence in the multidisciplinary team and that the consultant has no formal authority to prescribe tasks for them (Rowbottom 1978) and, on the other hand, of the importance of maintaining a close involvement with knowledge and issues affecting social work as a profession if their contribution to the team is to have any significance. Social work as a profession, meanwhile, would be impoverished without the contribution of the experience and ideas social workers have gained and developed from working with colleagues within multidisciplinary teams.

The tasks of the social worker on the bridge between the inpatient unit and the outside in many respects mirror those of the adolescent, who strives to incorporate what is best from within the family with what is best from friends, education and employment outside. While the adolescent may take flight from this tension either by retreating into the family or by leaving home abruptly and angrily, so the social worker may be tempted at times to seek to escape the discomfort of the bridge by, for example, either colluding with the nurses about the total impossibility of certain parents, or by joining with an outside social worker in criticising a decision about medication. But, just as the adolescent cannot progress without struggling with the tension of differing loyalties, so an adolescent unit cannot help its patients without taking on board the excitement and potential, as well as the irritation, of its ambivalent relationship with the outside world. However, unlike the adolescent, whose task it is to loosen ties with the family and become more independent, the social worker needs to remain firmly based both inside and outside the unit, as a member both of the multidisciplinary team and of the Social Services Department outside, despite the tensions intrinsic in such dual loyalty.

References and Further Reading

Brearley P, Black P, Gutridge P, Roberts G & Tarran E (1982) *Leaving Residential Care.* Residential Social Work Series. London: Tavistock

Bruggen P, Byng-Hall J & Pitt-Aikens T (1973) The reason for admission as a focus of work for an adolescent unit. *British Journal of Psychiatry,* **122,** 310-329

Bruggen P & O'Brian C (1984) Who solves the chronic problem: two professional family consultations. *Journal of Family Therapy,* **6**(2), 183-198

Bruggen P & Pitt-Aikens T (1975) Authority as a key factor in adolescent disturbance. *British Journal of Medical Psychology,* **48,** 153-159

Burck C (1978) A study of families' expectations and experiences of a child guidance clinic. *British Journal of Social Work,* **8**(2)

Eisenberg L (1975) The ethics of intervention – acting amidst ambiguity. *Journal of Child Psychology and Psychiatry,* **16,** 93-104

Gaylin W (ed) (1982) *Who Speaks for the Child?: The Problems of Proxy Consent.* London: Plenum Press

Gostin L (1975) *A Human Condition, Volume 1.* MIND Special Report

Lampen J (1981) Different perspectives. *Journal of Adolescence,* **4,** 199-209

Lask J & Lask B (1981) *Child Psychiatry and Social Work.* London: Tavistock Library of Social Work Practice

Laycock A L (1970) *Adolescence and Social Work.* Library of Social Work. London: Routledge & Kegan Paul

Rae M, Hewitt P & Hugill B (1982) *First Rights: A Guide to Legal Rights of Young People.* London: National Council for Civil Liberties

Reder P & Kraemer S (1980) Dynamic aspects of professional collaboration in child guidance referral. *Journal of Adolescence,* **3,** 165–173

Rowbottom R & Hey A (1978) *Organisation of Services for the Mentally Ill – A Working Paper.* London: Brunel Institute of Organisation and Social Studies

Winnicott D W (1971) *Playing and Reality.* London: Tavistock, 138–150

2 The Nursing of Adolescents

Michael Donnellan

Born and educated in the west of Ireland, I came to England in 1975 and began my career in nursing with three years' training as a psychiatric student nurse at Springfield Hospital, London, a large general psychiatric hospital, where I qualified as a Registered Mental Nurse (RMN) in 1978.

An interest in child and adolescent development and disorders led me to undertake the Joint Board of Clinical Nursing Studies course in Child and Adolescent Psychiatric Nursing at the Bethlem Royal Hospital and the Maudsley Hospital. On completion of the course I worked as a charge nurse at the Adolescent Unit, where I became interested in family therapy. I then trained in Family and Marital Therapy at the Institute of Family Therapy, London; this has proved invaluable to my work as a nurse.

———◆———

The Nursing Process

The adolescent in hospital needs to be looked after as an individual, yet is part of a family, and whilst in the adolescent unit is also part of its community. The nurse (who I will refer to as she in this chapter) has to be aware of these various dimensions of the adolescent's life; she has also to strike a balance between an informal approach and the more systematic approach of what has become known as the nursing process. In essence, this is based on a more formally organised procedure of assessment, goal-clarification, planned intervention and the evaluation of progress, and has replaced more haphazard aspects of nursing care. This systematic, goal-focused approach is quite compatible with other successful techniques in adolescent psychiatry, such as involving adolescent and family in making management plans and taking some responsibility for them, and in family review meetings where progress or lack of it is discussed with staff and new or renewed plans are made.

A common criticism of the nursing process is the time spent on the details of the work and in keeping records. However, we have been able to evolve methods which are practical and not too time-consuming, and which preserve for patients and staff the advantages of a properly organised approach. Nor have we found the introduction of the nursing process incompatible with the friendly informality between staff and patients which is another component of the unit's milieu.

Aspects of the Milieu

An effective, therapeutic milieu is intense and involving. Inevitably the nurse will come to be seen as a surrogate parent, and must be aware of the risk of seeming to undermine the role and authority of the adolescent's parents, a situation which can readily arise in the circumstances which lead to admission to hospital. The nurse must be aware of this tendency in herself, as well as being perceived in this way by adolescent and family. The nurse, in close liaison with the social worker or other family worker, may have to work quite hard to counter this impression, and emphasise instead that the parents have used their authority, responsibility and care for their child to seek psychiatric help and share responsibility with the nursing staff on a temporary basis. The closeness of the relationship between the nurse and the adolescent is an essential part of nursing, out of which should come effective therapeutic change. Managing this relationship does not come easily, and part of the challenge is remembering the parents' role. Often many nurses have themselves not long left their own adolescence and issues of becoming over-involved and questions of transference and counter-transference can present problems; one outcome may be identification with the adolescent against 'bad' parents. It is for such reasons that supervision of this aspect of nursing is so important. Such supervision can come either directly from other nurses in supervision sessions and weekly nurses' groups, or from other members of the team. Traditionally, supervision has often tended to come low on the list of priorities, but it must be seen as a necessary part of the nurse's development and education as well as underpinning good practice. Supervision in nursing has tended to be hierarchical, but I feel that a mixture of this system with peer consultation is a more progressive approach, augmented by similar joint work with members of other disciplines.

The ward of the adolescent unit is constantly undergoing change. Its physical, psychological and social maintenance as a 'holding' environment, providing stability without becoming rigid and institutionalised, is a crucial part of the nursing task. In order to create a milieu which itself can develop while being strong enough for the adolescent's development, the nurse must work with the wider team as well as with the adolescents, who themselves use and yet are part of the environment.

The organisation of the material aspects of the setting is most important. Such practicalities as food, warmth, comfort, safety, decoration, toys and games need to be attended to. But as well as the creation of this physical milieu, the 'meta milieu' is of equal importance; one follows from the other. This meta milieu emerges out of a well-structured, well-run, safe, secure and stimulating environment and takes into account the hidden agendas of the ward, those unspoken attitudes, beliefs, fears, annoyances and wishes which soon develop in any close community.

The nursing of adolescents includes dealing with the small issues of everyday living on the ward. Interactions are occurring all the time and the manner in which the nurse deals with them is a part of her skill in helping the adolescent patient deal with personal and interpersonal difficulties, change and growth. Because of the closeness and the intimate nature of the nurse–patient relationship over prolonged periods, the nurse has this task and opportunity much more directly than other members of the care team, and more frequently has to decide which to use and emphasise to make a point. For example, two adolescents differ about which programme to watch on television: this difference quickly spirals to become a much larger issue for those involved, resulting in harsh words and violence. The two are brought together and the problem of the outburst sorted out; but while an interim 'sorting-out' needs to happen, the incident deserves also to be examined carefully and in depth. If made a wider issue it can be used more effectively. The daily ward group run by the nurses is used to discuss why the incident might have happened, how it happened, and how it was resolved. Other adolescents in the group are invited to comment on how they view the incident and ways in which they might have dealt with it.

It is with such small issues that some of the nurse's most important therapeutic work is done, and how the nursing staff manage (and are seen to manage) such fragments of the community's day profoundly influences the whole milieu.

Rules and Boundaries

Every household has its rules. There must be times for getting up and going to bed, bed-making, breakfast, work, school, play, with a sense of security in the knowledge that no matter what happens (differences, damage, challenging of the rules) the structure will stand up to these assaults and remain intact. Yet although it is important to hold to a structure it is equally important to be flexible in the face of changing circumstances so that movement can occur for the sake of individual adolescents and for the group as a whole. The adolescents need the security of knowing that their distress, outbursts and challenges will be held within the psychological limits formed by the ward and the milieu; indeed an important factor in the decision to admit a boy or a girl is how much the boundaries of the unit may have to withstand heavy assault.

Two tools, the milieu and the nursing process, make up the primary foundation of nursing but, of course, there are many other ways through which the nurse promotes change and growth. Here, I think, there is a fundamental difference between nursing and practically all other professions (teaching is a possible exception); the nurse lives with, looks after and treats her patients all more or less at the same time. Thus there are both formal and informal roles; a nurse might be someone who accompanies a patient on an outing, plays a game of football, or goes camping, yet at another time she is a confidante or may be the adolescent's therapist.

These different roles can cause confusion in the adolescent, and in the nurse, too. Indeed, professional colleagues may develop a blurred vision of the nurse's function. It is difficult to avoid some areas of potential confusion, and to try too hard to do so could lead to an overconscientious, rigid, excluding attitude in a variety of legitimate nursing activities. What is important is to be aware of possible areas of confusion and be prepared to discuss them when and where appropriate. Perceptive supervision and planning, too, can ensure that particularly valuable work is not undermined. Thus, a nurse taking part in a particularly difficult piece of family work may not be the right person to accompany the boy or girl on an outing.

The Nurse and the Family

Only one member of the family – the 'identified patient' – is admitted to the unit. As mentioned earlier, it is important that the nurse does not lose sight of the family systems and the meanings and implications of separation, admission and of the family's continuing functioning and role. There is also likely to be a two-edged issue concerning the authority of the family and the authority of the nurse. In order that this be faced and resolved careful negotiation between the nurse, the patient and the family is necessary. Paradoxically, entry to hospital as an inpatient may for some adolescents and their families be quite a powerful message that the adolescent is now an individual in his or her own right, and not just a child. The question of including or not including the rest of the family (or other significant people) in the treatment programme is a most important issue, calling for early discussion and regular review. Certainly the family will always need to be involved in some way, but whether it be by just simply exchanging information or involving them in the decision making process depends on the individual adolescent's case. Characteristically, the lives of the young people we admit are often chaotic, with divided families and uncertain parental responsibilities, with community workers already involved, and with statutory legislation (eg. care orders) invoked or contemplated. Nonetheless, questions of authority, responsibility and consent must still be carefully negotiated and clarified.

> Philip, aged 13 years, is admitted after having become completely beyond the control of his family. He is aggressive and has temper tantrums almost hourly, hitting his mother and smashing-up the household when asked to do anything. Philip cannot, or will not, control himself and he is referred to the adolescent unit for assessment. Things have gone so far that arrangements are made for Philip to be admitted.
>
> His parents are immediately relieved, but it is important that this much-needed relief is not confused with being relieved of responsibility and authority.
>
> Whether Philip behaves better in the unit or not, the nursing staff take care to involve his family (parents and siblings) at every stage of assessment and in the treatment programme. As with all adolescents admitted, a family worker has been allocated to the case (in this instance a social worker), meeting the family every week. Thus, the immediate caring team becomes triangular: parents and adolescent; family worker; nurses.
>
> On meeting the family before admission it becomes evident that the parents need to do much work to regain their authority. It is made clear to Philip that the unit is acting on his parents' behalf, at their request and with their approval. From a nursing viewpoint,

this is achieved by involving the parents in deciding on and applying sanctions and by teaching them more effective methods of handling difficulties. As progress is made, the parents properly take credit for gains made, although they may well find this hard to do.

Formal family therapeutic sessions take place weekly, and family review meetings every few weeks. Meanwhile, for the nurses, daily contact with Philip's parents is indicated in order that problems which present may be 'handed back' to the parents as the people in charge of Philip. This daily contact and 'handing back' throws up all sorts of issues and dilemmas for both the nurse and the family. The nurse's skill is in not undermining the parental effort and authority; the work must be maintained as a cooperative effort rather than a competition over who can best control.

The right balance and a phased handing back, with positive connotation of the parents' competence, was successfully employed in order to get Philip home again.

Mandy, a 16-year-old girl, illustrates different aspects of the nurse's role. Mandy had very severe anxiety symptoms for some three years, related to epilepsy. Two other adolescent services had tried to help but were unsuccessful. On meeting Mandy's family at a pre-admission visit to their home, her mother and father both proved to be very anxious and intensely involved with her to an unhelpful degree; it was clear from the outset that in this case some disengagement between the parents and Mandy would almost certainly be needed to help her and her parents to make a fresh start. However, for the nurse to take upon herself the responsibility for making a unilateral recommendation about admission seemed inappropriate, and perhaps disastrous to the progress of management, if not to the family among whom very mixed feelings were powerful.

For Mandy's benefit her parents needed to be involved in order that they might learn how not to be so over-involved; their anxieties had to be heeded and concentrated upon and slow but steady moves made towards creating trust between the nurse, the patient and family.

On this basis, the decision for a period of separation, with Mandy in the unit for a time, came as much from the family as from the nurse undertaking this preliminary work, and their decision in itself was a significant first therapeutic step, as well as being 'safer' than a decision made by a professional worker.

In the first example, nursing and family therapy were kept separate, the latter to a considerable extent helping to sustain the former. In the second example the nursing task came much closer to family therapy.

How far can the adolescent's nurse be involved in family therapy? In my experience, good, effective, therapeutic nursing of the adolescent and attempts by the nurse to become directly involved in family therapy do not mix easily, and may indeed prove antithetic to each other. Not only does the nurse's role become blurred if she attempts this work but the child and parents may become confused. This is not to say that nurses should never become involved in family work, and indeed many do so very effectively; but it is important that a clear role and purpose is defined for the nurse/family worker, and in general it is best if this nurse is not the primary nurse for the adolescent's day-to-day management. Again, supervision, and ideally joint supervision shared between a family therapy and a nursing supervisor, helps to clarify tasks and monitor progress.

The Nurse and Teamwork

To achieve 'good enough' unity in the nursing team is hard work, and sometimes links break down and miscommunication and rivalry creep in. It is my belief that the traditional relative isolation of the nurse, somewhat reluctant to admit to seniors when help and support are needed, and even more so in relation to other disciplines, contributes to this. It may also be that other professionals in multidisciplinary work have not felt themselves to be close enough to the nurse to offer help. This may be due to caution over crossing boundaries and intruding into the nurse's sphere or, indeed, to failure by the nurse to accept the wider team concept. Nurses have been quick to point out to other professionals whenever it seemed that they were trying to organise nursing for nurses, and in my view this has led to a gap between nurses and the rest; fortunately, nursing has moved away from its former isolated position and this makes the concept of multidisciplinary support more realistic and attainable. However, it does not come easily and has to be worked for. By support in this context I mean mutual working, good liaison, both separate and shared supervision and teaching and common staff support groups.

I have already mentioned that the adolescent in the unit needs a structure; it is important that the nurses' programme should also have structure and organisation and include a group where issues such as their closeness with the patient, or feeling that they are not being listened to, or are undervalued, can be worked on with the rest of the team. They will find such feelings familiar to others.

An effective and unified team will face such issues, acknowledge differences and place their differences in perspective. Nurses, doctors, social workers, teachers, psychologists, occupational therapists and anyone else who is part of the care team, need to have their own aims and strategies, and sometimes these will be different and perhaps in conflict. Intense, anxiety-making work can sometimes force conflict, or result in disciplines drawing apart.

Peter, a 15-year-old boy, was admitted following many serious and determined suicide attempts. Like Mandy, he had been an inpatient for a long time in another unit before treatment had fallen through. He presented a challenge to the whole team, but the nurses took on the central role of keeping Peter alive, in effect providing a life-support system. They expressed this intensity to the rest of the staff by raising such questions as – can we hold this difficult situation? Do we need to detain him on a Section of the Mental Health Act? Is there a need for medication? For transfer to a more secure environment? Perhaps even discharge to yet another hospital? Initially there was an increasing tendency for the nurses to carry all the burden; Peter could not be safely supervised away from the unit, and, later, could not be supervised so closely in the school. The responsibility the nurses took was willingly and efficiently assumed but operated against sharing feelings and responsibilities with other disciplines, except by the above questions. What these questions generated, most importantly, was the explicit response from other staff that Peter could not be managed without taking risks, and that excessive containment and protection could well inhibit that growth that would give Peter a chance of a safe future. The intense 'containing' process now began to reverse, with nurses sharing with others the work with Peter, the responsibility and the anxiety, and achieved a safe balance between protection and overprotection that was as important for the staff as it proved to be for Peter.

Conclusion

I believe that the role of the nurse and the practice of nursing is moving away from the boundaries that have been built around it over the years. It is important not to disregard what has been good in nursing in the past, but the nurse now has to embrace new developments, and these include moving with patients into the wider community outside the hospital institution. In this process the nursing profession has to learn from other professions, and also has much to teach. The new General Nursing Council Syllabus of Training for Mental Nurses (1982), for example, provides a more radical approach to the training of psychiatric nurses, and gives more attention to adolescents and their problems and to the family. While the numbers involved in adolescent nursing may be small, the problems and approaches in this field have wider relevance within the whole of nursing.

References and Further Reading

Barker P (1981) *Basic Family Therapy*. London: Granada, pp 21–40; 167–176

Burr J & Andrews J (1981) *Nursing the Psychiatric Patient*. London: Baillière Tindall, pp 248–256

Fagin C M (ed) (1974) *Readings in Child and Adolescent Psychiatric Nursing*. St Louis, Mo: C V Mosby Co

Irving S (1983) *Basic Psychiatric Nursing*. London: W B Saunders Co

Kratz C (ed) (1979) *The Nursing Process*. London: Baillière Tindall

McFarlane J & Castledine G (1982) *A Guide to the Practice of Nursing Using the Nursing Process*. London: C V Mosby Co

Robinson L (1977) *Psychiatric Nursing as a Human Experience*. London: W B Saunders Co, pp 390–420

Wilkinson T R (1983) *Child and Adolescent Psychiatric Nursing*. Oxford: Blackwell Scientific Publications, pp 173–273

3 The Adolescent Unit School: Education and Therapy

Brian Molloy

I returned to this country from Zimbabwe fifteen years ago with a training and background that included history, sociology and education, and experience in remedial work with physically handicapped children. Perhaps it was this unusual combination of interests that led me towards the field in which I could find room for my various enthusiasms: psychiatry. I was appointed to a vacancy in the school in the Adolescent Unit of Bethlem Royal and Maudsley Hospitals, and began a most exciting and rewarding career, experiencing for the first time work in a psychiatric team. I must have been a square peg in a square hole, for soon I was offered the post of acting deputy. The opportunity to complete training in my chosen branch of teaching came when I was seconded to the Institute of Education, University of London, to take the Diploma in the Education of Maladjusted Children. For my dissertation I chose the subject 'The interprofessional perspectives between teachers and nurses working in psychiatric units'. After this course I was appointed Headteacher to what was then the new school at Beech House Adolescent Unit in Kent. During this time I had become an active member of the Association for the Psychiatric Study of Adolescents (APSA), of which I was later to become secretary and then chairman.

History

The year 1944 marks the coming of age of Special Education in Great Britain, though, it must be admitted, it was a long time a-growing! The need for special provision for the blind and deaf had been realised before the end of the eighteenth century. Physically handicapped and epileptic children were provided for in the nineteenth century, but the disturbed and the maladjusted youngster was not considered to have special needs until almost half way through the twentieth century. Child psychiatrists in the early days had to admit their patients to hospital to provide them with what the Underwood Report described as 'Planned Environmental Therapy'.

Since the beginning of the century some inspired pioneers, aware that problems existed for young people who could not cope with traditional schools founded on ideas of competition, subject teaching and corporal punishment, had broken away and set up progressive schools and communities. These establishments differed from each other as they depended for their existence on the beliefs of the founders. Otto Shaw introduced selfgovernment when he opened Redhill School as he believed in shared responsibility; George Lyward, the mystic, removed all pressures at Fynchden Manor and surrounded his boys with a loving, creative atmosphere; Leila Rendal founded the Caldecott Community to meet the needs of refugee children during the war, and it was so successful that she kept it open to meet the needs of deprived children when the war was over.

By 1944 it was imperative that the Department of Education and Science (DES) should respond to the ever-growing needs of disturbed children and adolescents, and the problem known as maladjustment was acknowledged in an Act which defined 11 categories of handicap for which authorities would make provision in special or ordinary schools. With the Educational (Handicapped Children) Act 1970, local education authorities assumed responsibility for mentally handicapped children (previously the responsibility of health authorities) and for the first time all children were considered educable. The report of the Warnock Committee, 1978, and the Education Act 1981 are manifestations in statute of changes in thinking about the special educational needs of children and young people, and of the way in which provision should be made for them. There is now much alternative provision for children with different problems, and the Act advocates full integration into the community whenever possible.

Schools and Hospital Units

Adolescent units grew out of the response to the need for better work with young people exhibiting emotional problems; the educational provision came as an afterthought. This was apparent in so much as the physical provision for this education was often a backroom – even a bathroom – on the ward.

Educational provision may take many forms: part-time attendance at both the unit and outside schools; fulltime attendance at either the unit or outside school. An inpatient unit may have no educational provision on the unit premises, and patients are expected to attend nearby schools on a fulltime basis. Some day patient units expect part-time attendance at the unit school *and* outside school. The size of the educational provision on the unit premises varies. DES Circular 4/73 recommends a staffing ratio of a Head plus 7 or 8 teachers for 30 children. Teaching staff holiday patterns vary throughout the country; teachers cannot be absent for many weeks in the year without upsetting the team. An indication of the unity of medical and educational staff is sometimes shown when the school remains open throughout the year.

Each adolescent unit has its own ethos and structure, and many questions arise before we can understand the position of education in each unit. The answers to these questions should be included in the total aims of the unit. Why are the young people in or attending these units? Where does their educational programme fit in? The existence of a school in a unit, with governors, headteacher, deputy and staff, will have given the school a great deal of importance. The school is thereby placed in a somewhat contradictory position. Unlike a special school admitting pupils with emotional and behavioural problems which affect learning, the headteacher does not have the right of admission and discharge. The young people are admitted as patients and not pupils. How far the headteacher and governors can influence matters of policy depends on the relationship between hospital staff and those employed by the education authority.

The Headteacher

Winston Churchill once remarked that the headteacher of an English school had more power in his own domain than that vested in a Prime Minister. This is not the case in a hospital school. The school depends on the goodwill of all partners in the multidisciplinary team if it is to function effectively. The headteacher has a major part to play in facilitating the use of this goodwill to ensure stimulation and success for both staff and patients. In doing so the headteacher will have to weave a diplomatic way through the multidisciplinary maze. It is to be hoped that individual personalities do not play the greatest part in working for or against co-operation between individual professionals and disciplines, but often there can be a subordination of working relationships to personal issues.

The headteacher acts as both educational consultant and manager. A colleague once said that a headteacher is expected to make dynamic, executive, administrative decisions – and act with authority! In fact the headteacher can only make decisions within the school. If he wishes to implement an activity or policy which affects work with patients outside the classroom, he has to act in liaison with other professionals, and may well find that the multidisciplinary decision-making process can inhibit creativity.

In other schools the headteacher has more time to carry out administrative and consultative duties; for most headteachers of psychiatric units schools, frequent attendance at unit meetings is expected. If there is more than one consultant psychiatrist and more than one building to divide one's attention (eg. children's department and adolescent unit), attending such meetings can exceed 60% of one's time, and priorities have to be decided. Attendance at school and educational meetings and case conference have to be priorities. The school's meetings should serve a threefold purpose:
  (i)   the reporting and planning of school programmes for individual patients. Record keeping must be purposeful and in line with future planning,
  (ii)   administration, policy making and sharing of information. These meetings can always include elements of in-service training, and
  (iii) informal sensitivity type meetings to enhance a better working relationship between the members of the teaching staff.

Much time is spent in liaison with other professionals in the educational field. As part of an informal 10-year review at one adolescent unit, it was realised that the headteacher had had contact with more than 215 different educational establishments, for example at initial referral, or at placement on discharge. This involved approaching not only headteachers and staff but educational welfare officers, psychologists, and a variety of educational administrators, to deal with patients' educational needs. This 'educational' contact did not include contact with careers officers and employers. All this leaves very little time for a headteacher to see patients, and he needs really good staff who can work together and carry out the aims of the school. Within the unit, in my experience, one works more often with the charge nurses and sisters than with other members of the team.

Individual Programming

Before admission, it is useful if the headteacher contacts the patient's school, school psychologist and education welfare officer to discuss educational issues, and to check whether or not the parent school is offering to reintegrate the patient in due course.

Admission policies vary from unit to unit, but an example of good practice is where on admission the patient spends some time first on the ward, before attending school. During these first days the patient is assessed by various members of the team. This includes an assessment undertaken by the school of attainments, skills, and interests. This forms the basis on which a patient's individual programme can be formulated, but with the medical programme having priority.

In some psychiatric units the daily programme is an automatic process; every patient attends set functions – therapy or school – at set times, and this allows minimal scope for meeting individual needs. In many establishments 'treatment' takes place before and after school time, and in between the patients trot off to school in various shades of motivation. Is this automatic burst of one thing or another really efficient in terms of treatment, time and cost effectiveness? Individual programming should include all other aspects of multidisciplinary working in order to be effective.

The role of the nurse in school is something special. Nurses are not teachers, nor extensions of teachers, nor ancillary help to the school staff. It may be that a nurse can share with a teacher the security of his or her relationship with a patient; it may be appropriate for a nurse and teacher to work out a programme together. It may be necessary for that nurse to observe the patient working with the teacher, perhaps available within the school building but not actually in the class. This can reassure a patient, particularly after a patient has spent some time on the ward as part of the treatment programme and is beginning to reintegrate into school.

The Teacher and the Team

All too often the role of the teacher in the multidisciplinary team becomes too blurred. Some blurring is appropriate, but it should come about through a skilful use of subject teaching, rather than through 'dabbling' with psychotherapy. Surely there is more than enough work for each discipline to undertake and so employ their own precise and exact skills. This does not exclude the adults dropping their particular roles and joining together as adults in 'activities' with the patients. For a reduction of tension between disciplines, role definition is essential, unless everyone is doing everything under equal conditions of service!

Equally essential to the reduction of tension is that the adults should be adults together. This implies very clear planning between the disciplines and especially between the nurses and teachers. Although the emphasis may be on formal programming, the notion of fun for fun's sake is vital. It may be the first experience of fun, or the first for a long time, for many patients. Fun activities undertaken by nurses or teachers during the school day have been considered a poor use of time; I would argue strongly against this.

The school also provides various learning experiences in groups. Patients can be prepared and entered for examinations, which always receives applause. Patients feel achievement not just in sitting an exam, but in receiving realistic evidence of success. Success for the less academic can be found in many other areas such as drama productions, and in sports and gymnastic exercises. Learning can be stimulating *and* fun, and therefore ego satisfying. In turn, the new found confidence promotes closer relationships with authority figures.

From a teacher's point of view some of the joys of teaching in a psychiatric unit arise from the stimulation of working with patients on a short term basis. At the closing session of an APSA Annual Conference, George Lyward spoke about adolescents being both 'wilful' and 'soulful'. The joy is in finding the soul and enabling it to be revealed safely and securely, and so allow a will to continue to make further progress. In both wilful and soulful are the words full; when things are full, they usually require emptying, and replacing with something good and new. It is in the creation and use of teaching methods and programmes during short stay that one can fully appreciate the Lyward philosophy. There is also pleasure in working in close cooperation with a cross section of professionals and ancillary staff; their different approaches make for mental refreshment and challenge and this taps and stretches staff potential. A strange pleasure comes, too, from working with the unpredictable, and being flexible enough to respond. Because of shift and sessional systems and working commitments, one is never quite sure which staff are going to be on duty on any one day. Each day brings a refreshing start, although sometimes lack of continuity may be frustrating. Finally, much of the joy of work in a multidisciplinary team is through working with different people as individuals, rather than with different professional groups.

Education and Therapy

Many members of the multidisciplinary team look upon the school as being the only place in the unit primarily exercising normality. The school may offer such positive experiences to the patients but more important, or so it seems, the school has to be a positive experience for one's colleagues, and staff perceptions of the educational provision is fraught with expectations based on their own good and bad school experiences. Teachers need to be conscious of this, in making a contribution to the team which is both educational and therapeutic and consistent with each adolescent's overall programme, and which begins from a normal rather than clinical position.

Tasks for education and tasks for therapy have strong links. Most would agree that $2 + 2$ equals 4, practically as an automatic response, and that is normal. But the process used to reach such conclusions is seldom normal. Division and subtraction are something to do with sharing and giving away, addition and multiplication are to do with increases, and one can anticipate arithmetical problems related to emotional difficulties, for example in the inability of anorexic patients to undertake proper mentation with their total thinking absorbed by the notion of starving and food.

In the writer's pilot study into the relationship between encopresis and arithmetical attainment, it was observed that encopretics may have low arithmetical attainments. One could go further into considerations of the psychological nature of number and suggest that number is an anal subject. To some it is cold and aggressive, and is reliant on the use of computational logic in using the correct stimulus to equal the appropriate response. Encopresis can be considered as an aggressive act directed at an aspect of a patient's relationships. Daily experience has shown that encopretics tend to find number work very annoying. The best they seem to do is to produce sheets of digital smearing, usually stuck at a particular and very basic arithmetical process. It may be advisable for teachers to leave the teaching of number to encopretics well alone until such time that the patient begins to enjoy sharing activities with one other, and then with more than one person – peer or adult.

The same applies to the teaching of English – more especially to the teaching of reading. English is an oral subject. Many patients resist oral activities and some are unable to digest the academic offering. Of course there are those who merely gobble the offering and use it as a defence against appreciating its qualities, like some anorexics. Once again a different set of activities has to be employed to allow the patient to develop trust and security to release his emotions and so unblock the learning processes. Geography may not be undertaken well by those patients who experience a bad body image. An excessively well-built 14-year-old girl was struggling to meet the teacher's demands in a geography lesson. She was lying on top of the lockers in the classroom. On the teacher enquiring what she was doing, she said 'Geography'. On further enquiring what aspect of geography, she stated 'mountains' – obviously. A boy suffering from Tourette's syndrome undertook studying 'pre-pre-neolithic' in History and 'outer, outer solar systems' in Science. As he was enabled to come to terms with his problems, he progressed to Ancient Egypt and then later, to the modern world. Physical education involves body expression. One could wonder why it is that this lesson always seems to have non-participant pupils hanging around the edge? What do the inabilities of those less able bring out in those who are able, eg. PE teachers? What attitude does the teacher adopt to the pupil at such a time?

It is the subtle use of a special approach to normal teaching in these and other ways that gives the teacher special value in the multidisciplinary team.

Conclusion

From what has been said, clearly I hope that the aims of the school would be incorporated into the aims of the unit as a whole; but never should the multidisciplinary working relationship be taken for granted. From the moment one enters this specialised field of teaching one must be open to new ideas and be prepared to take every opportunity to assimilate experience and knowledge. It is hoped that teachers would endeavour to further their training through secondments, in-service courses, and Association (like APSA) study days and conferences.

The 1981 Act stresses special needs, and correctly so. However, courses are now being geared towards the special needs in the ordinary school. It is worrying that the study of patients' problems as taught in the psychiatric unit schools is being put aside. In understanding the dynamics of such patients/pupils one can gain useful insights into the behaviour and emotional lives of the pupils in the ordinary school. For example, with the current emphasis on community work, it seems appropriate to consider ways in which the school, as well as the unit as a whole, can act as a resource centre. The adolescent unit school could offer specialist services to outside educational establishments in the form of student placements, supervision of support units and special needs departments, liaison with special needs panels, and could take a lead in offering in-service training courses.

References and Further Reading

Axline V M (1966) *Dibs: In Search of Self*. Harmondsworth: Penguin Books
ACE (1981) Special Education Handbook: Education Act 1981. London: Contone Printers
Bridgeland M (1971) *Pioneer Work with Maladjusted Children*. London: Staples Press
Hegarty S & Pocklington K (1981) *Educating Pupils with Special Needs in the Ordinary School*. Walton-on-Thames: NFER/Nelson
Hegarty *et al* (1982) *Integration in Action*. Walton-on-Thames: NFER/Nelson
Salzberger-Wittenberg I (1983) *The Emotional Experience of Learning and Teaching*. London: Routledge & Kegan Paul

Sycamore A (1971) *Sebastian's. A Hospital School Experiment in Therapeutic Education*. London: Longmans

Warnock H M (1978) Report of the Committee of Enquiry into the Education of Handicapped Children and Young People. London: HMSO

Acknowledgement

My thanks to Mrs D O'Connor for sharing this and many other tasks.

The Adolescent Unit
Edited by Derek Steinberg
© 1986 D. Steinberg

4 Music in the Education of the Disturbed Adolescent

Deirdre Page

My employment in a school within a psychiatric unit for adolescents was almost an accident, since my interest lay with mentally handicapped patients and their musical potential. Since the age of sixteen I had run bands of singing and percussion playing with mentally handicapped children and adults, and while at Homerton College I worked with a group of physically handicapped children boarding at a school near Cambridge. From this work I came to believe that music was within everyone, but for some the desire to express it was too inhibited.

I was in my early twenties when I started working at Bethlem. Mrs D O'Connor, the headmistress at the time, selected her teachers with an emphasis on specialist qualities rather than specialist qualifications. I had energy and enthusiasm to offer as well as teaching qualifications and thus I started work, learning as I went along. I knew of no other music specialist doing similar work and developed a style of my own which led people to tend to call me a music therapist. I call myself a music teacher, as a teacher will encourage and stretch an individual, using the pupil's own talent as a basis for self-expression; my perception of a therapist is someone who may use self-expression in one of the arts as the basis for a psychotherapeutic relationship, used to relieve disorder or overcome handicap with the technical quality of the work done of little importance.

———◆———

The Adolescent Unit School at Bethlem is a most inspired building in which to work. Carefully planned to create natural grouping in its curved seating and stairway, its classrooms are warm and inviting, each one divided into three sections for the lone worker, small group and main group.

There was no music teacher when the school was designed, so there was no room sufficiently insulated to save the rest of the school from hearing every bang and crash emitting from my lessons. Physical education, I discovered, took place largely in the main hospital gymnasium and on the football pitch, and it was with very little subtlety that I requisitioned the school's own gymnasium and turned it into a music hall. Although rather large for music-making in small groups, it is ideal for uninhibited exploratory work and the courage and trust that this needs. The initiated rush ahead to have a foretaste of the larger instruments; the more reluctant, cautious ones straggle in, taking a seat quietly, some hoping not to be noticed, others that they will be given the necessary encouragement to risk exploring sound. When the door is closed, the school and the unit seem far away and music-making has all our attention.

I try to give every member of the school some kind of musical experience although it is not a compulsory subject. Often an adolescent will arrive full of prejudice about music, expecting perhaps to have to play 'London's Burning' yet again on the recorder or to learn boring old notation and theory from a blackboard. I am excited when I have a pupil with this image of school music as it gives me a chance to invite the boy or girl to try a new experience which will challenge that prejudice.

In an environment where attitudes, feelings and behaviour are constantly in focus, I think it important to give the adolescent an opportunity to divert and use a non-verbal form of communication, and one which will not be mistaken for a 'treatment'. Music is one of the arts offering this; it is a part of every one of us. The body's mechanics provide rhythms and beats and there is melody and harmony in the natural sounds we make. Music is a universal experience that we can all share in, and of course a cultural inheritance too.

Adolescents are cautious of musical improvisation; they think it might be childish. To enable me to take them back to this simple beginning I have good quality instruments and always insist upon the utmost respect for them, although this does not exclude using them in extraordinary ways. Ideally, there should be a wide choice of sound and I have found a few African and Indian percussion instruments have added variety to the usual orchestral percussion selection.

I begin with small groups that start with the most basic primeval forms of aural (and sometimes oral) communication. The most important factor at the beginning is a trust that the group will not laugh at the individual's contribution. Often I start with a frivolous word or sound game which gives the pupils a chance to laugh, and this is followed by simple and more serious exercises employing the same sounds. For example, the pupils choose a number between one and eight and select an instrument or oral noise of their choice. While the eight beats are silently counted, each member contributes his or her noise on the chosen number. This can be expanded to take in an instrumental *and* oral noise per person and more than one note played per beat.

Communication being vital, I always have the group in a circle so everyone can see each other. When each member has chosen an instrument we begin work on our eye contact by playing sound games round the circle, and the sound is passed around at random as one player focusses on another. Simplicity must be maintained and emotional investment brought in only slowly and sparingly. It quickly becomes apparent who is going to need encouragement to work in this medium and who adapts naturally to it. Music should be a positive experience and in these improvised groups no sincere effort is good or bad.

Self-control is more often than not something to work towards with my pupils; the power of silence is unknown to many of them. Silence is part of sound and music, which are the richer for their controlled contrasts.

So, having included oral noises in the games or exercises from the beginning, strange noises from the mouth or throat become part of making music. It also dispenses with the need for giggly raspberry-blowing as expressions of misbehaviour and embarrassment, since these noises conform exactly to what I ask for. The amount of time spent on these games and exercises varies from group to group but with a good group I would have two or three sessions of them before bringing in a more exacting task.

Another exercise is to interpret the Elements in an abstract and atmospheric manner, giving the pupils an opportunity to express moods not dissimilar from their own, but with much safer labels such as storm, avalanche, rain, sunshine or flood. I may develop these ideas into a project and ask the adolescents to create a notational system of their own using colour or symbols to incorporate the volume, speed and shape of sound. As we become more impressionist, so the score can become more widely interpreted (Fig. 4.1).

This is often a good point to bring in conventional scoring and combine the idea of an individual's creativity with the reliable reproduction of an idea. Learning to read music is much easier when it is seen to be logical, and I encourage more traditional instrumental tuition for musically-awakened pupils by introducing, for example, the piano, flute, clarinet, classical guitar or recorder.

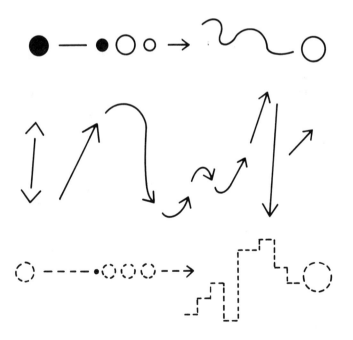

Fig. 4.1 Informal scoring for two-part playing with two slightly different volumes. (pitch indicated in between)

Mainstream schoolteachers envy the size of class with which I am able to work, and this is indeed an advantage. It is possible to spend much more time on a pupil's gifts or difficulties when working with a group of between two and eight people, and while the opportunity to work alone with one boy or girl is an uncommon privilege for an ordinary class music teacher, it is frequent for me. But there is a disadvantage too: I am unable to build up a choir or orchestra and give my pupils that valuable, traditional experience of performing a well-rehearsed piece, becoming more accomplished each year as the group progresses; this is something I miss.

The guitar is a very popular instrument and I encourage my pupils to learn it. Our Education Authority has kindly loaned the school several guitars as well as our larger percussion instruments, and these stimulate the adolescents' interest in singing their own type of songs or making their own type of music out of school-time and amongst themselves. For young people not so interested in the classical guitar or folk-music, I have a pop group for rhythm guitar, bass guitar, electric organ and drums, all of which instruments are on loan. As an accomplished performance is an invaluable boost to a pupil's confidence, I am always on the look-out for music that sounds impressive but when broken down into parts is basic and easily learned. When pupils hear that they can make music that sounds accomplished, they can tackle skills and techniques with more determination and confidence because they no longer have to prove that they are not hopeless.

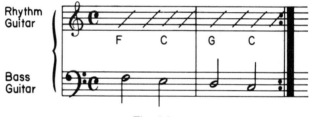

Fig. 4.2

To show how to produce an easy and good sound, I demonstrate with Simon and Garfunkel's '59th Street Bridge Song' (Feelin' Groovy). We listen to the real thing on tape and pick out the details, noting that there are no drums and no organ. It is a two-part song with a repeated four-chord pattern throughout. I am no drummer and depend upon the skill of the individual who is keen enough to pick up the rhythmic pattern himself; fortunately there is always someone able to do this, and so a drumming part is added. The bass guitarist plays the simple pattern illustrated (Fig. 4.2) while the rhythm guitarist strums the chord pattern and the keyboard player plays the chords similarly, or according to his capability. And so, based on a one chord-pattern, it is possible to build up a complete performance and then add the voice parts, as shown in Fig. 4.3.

From this we are able to move on to songs that have repetitive chord progressions, but with added complications such as a different middle section. An example of this is the old chestnut from the fifties called 'Dream' which uses 'the student vamp' that so many children learn (C major, A minor, F major, G major) and, more up to date, 'Walking on the Moon' by Police (D minor, C major).

I frequently find that pupils are more willing to be chastised and rebuked by their peers than risk using their voices to sing. The singing voice is an extremely personal attribute which many people find too exposing to use in spite of it being a musical instrument we all possess. People often describe themselves as tone deaf but I have never met such a person, and I revel in the pleasure given to someone who has believed that he could not sing in tune and finds after a few sessions that he can, and does it well. Of course, there are people who do not listen to the sound their voice makes, and as the ear is not attending to the voice, the sound is not in tune. Some of my pupils are very unaware of their bodies and minds in relation to others, and are consequently un-aware of vocal disharmony, too, a problem often consistent with their other difficulties.

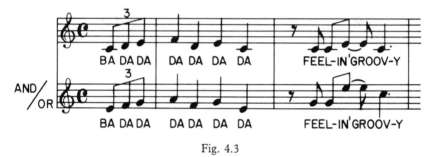

Fig. 4.3

When Patricia, who was electively mute, was first admitted to our unit, she was extremely keen to play the drums. It was fortuitous that one of our nursing staff was a keen drummer. He taught her all he knew in about ten lessons, and after he left she continued to teach herself with a book on the art of drumming. She had played the guitar at her previous school and was obviously musically talented. Her music lessons included drumming, guitar and improvisation. She had used her voice in a percussive manner in improvisation, and alongside her improvement in speaking I was able to coax her to sing. Her speaking voice sounded loud, forced and lacked intonation, and likewise her singing voice was a monotone, sounding lifeless and quite inexpressive. We abandoned the guitar and practised moving the voice from low to high pitch, holding notes, stopping and repeating the same note. In a remarkably short time Patricia was concentrating her ears to hear the sound from her throat, and we were soon singing together with the guitars again. But her speaking voice continued to be loud and unmusical.

The singer who has given me the most pleasure in my work is Beth; a 'strange child' was her own description of herself. She was unable to communicate easily and got muddled and frightened by people and events around her. She would try most earnestly in all her general lessons and could often be seen pacing around the unit with her elbows dug into her waist and her clenched hands against each cheek. When she would come to sing in the Music Hall, her hands would drop to her sides,

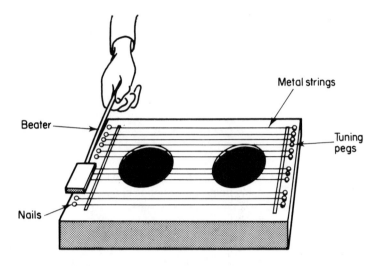

Chordal Dulcimer

Fig. 4.4

and as she sang her arms would rise and with open hands and wide open mouth she would pour her body and soul into her voice. She always sang a song in the key which I originally taught her, and showed enormous enjoyment. She could make up her own songs too, about the dilemma of her life, and also learned arias by Handel, which she sang exquisitely. It seemed a good idea to teach Beth the guitar so that she could accompany herself in her own time, and extend her periods of unwinding and relaxing through music. In fact her co-ordination and dexterity were so poor that I had to think of other accompanying instruments that were less complicated. When I was seventeen, I had attended a ten-day 'Music for the Handicapped' Course at Dartington College of Arts, and had made a Chordal Dulcimer (Fig. 4.4). This is a rectangular box, approximately 18″ by 6″ by 2″ with twelve strings tuned in four groups of three, making the chords of C Major, F Major, G Major and D Major. With a flat beater striking the triads there was an instant accompaniment. Beth was used to the colour-coding I had used in group music-making and so I gave her the dulcimer with a book of songs she knew, which I had colour-coded. She took them with her when she moved on to live in a Rudolf Steiner Community.

Once or twice a year we hold a folk evening where the patients and unit staff all gather in the school and perform vocal and instrumental pieces for one another. This gives the unit a chance to perform and risk exposing its talents. The patients often need encouragement and much rehearsal in order to feel sufficient confidence to perform.

Each October the Maudsley and Bethlem Royal Hospitals celebrate their Founders, beginning with a service in the Chapel. It has become an annual event for the adolescents to join with adult patients and staff in a choir which I lead. Often in cassock and surplice, we perform a different choral piece from Bach to Elgar, or a four-part negro spiritual or even a suitable excerpt from a musical. This gives the adolescents a taste of public performance and gives me some idea of the pupils willing to perform at Christmas when the biggest entertainment that the unit provides takes place.

For the past thirty years a pantomime or show has been produced each Christmas; 1981 was an exception, when we felt that it would not be of use to the group of patients we had at the time. In the 1950s it was in traditional English pantomime style with the script written in verse. In the 1960s a looser, more improvised style developed.

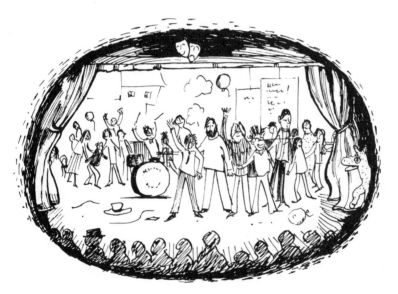

Pantomime has become a project in which the whole unit takes part. The patients continue their treatment programmes while a new priority is brought into their lives. We endeavour to include every patient on the unit in the show, by acting, making scenery, props, and costumes, and with good relationships between staff and a lot of enthusiasm, each individual patient has the chance to take on a character or role and discover unknown resources and new-found confidence. These annual shows are an excellent opportunity to make bullies into heroes or heroines, the 'good' child a baddy, and those who cannot see themselves as good, attractive or of interest, the chance to be so on stage. A great sense of togetherness and mutual encouragement develops, characteristically around a core of adolescents who fervently believe in the show; this keeps the whole thing together so that when doubts creep in, in true theatrical tradition the 'show-must-go-on' element prevails. There is then on The Night the chance to show parents, friends and staff the well and normal part of themselves so often hidden by problems and ill-health. Frequently, the most surprised person is the patient, who only realises what he has achieved during and after the performance. It appears to be something treasured in the memories of the individual, for when past patients meet members of staff, they reminisce over their part in their particular show with great nostalgia.

In the cut-backs and economies of the present, I imagine that teachers and therapists of creative expression may seem an expensive luxury, yet I wonder how else this so well and normal part of the disordered or disabled young person can be brought out and used. In psychiatry, words are the main vehicle of expression and that which is unspoken is teased out or interpreted. There should always be room made for that other part of ourselves as whole people, the revelation of thought and emotion through the Arts whatever our state of mind. We can deny ourselves the privilege all too easily, and our patients more easily still.

References and Further Reading

Alvin J (1976) *Music for the Handicapped Child*. Oxford: Oxford University Press
Alvin J (1975) *Music Therapy* (Revised Edition). London: Hutchinson
Bailey P (1973) *They can make Music*. Oxford: Oxford University Press
Coate M (1964) *Beyond all Reason*. London: Constable
Coleman J (1964) *Music for Exceptional Children*. London: Sammy-Birchard
Copeland A (1952) *Music and Imagination*. Harvard University Press/Mentor Books
Finkelstein S W (1952) *How Music expresses Ideas*. London: Lawrence & Wishart
Thayer Gaston E (ed) (1968) *Music in Therapy*. New York: Collier Macmillan
McLaughlin T (1970) *Music and Communication*. London: Faber
Priestley M (1975) *Music Therapy in Action*. London: Constable
Roberts R (1965) *Musical Instruments Made to be Played*. London: Dryad
van de Wall W (1964) *Music in Hospitals*. New York: Russell Sage Foundation
Ward D (1972) *Sound Approaches for Slow Learners*. London: Bedford Square Press

The Adolescent Unit
Edited by Derek Steinberg
© 1986 D. Steinberg

5 Art in the Education of the Disturbed Adolescent

Jacqueline Merry

I was born in 1941 and educated at a convent school. I then lived in France and Canada and held a variety of jobs before becoming an art student in 1968. While doing the teachers' training course at Hornsey College I became involved in various special projects which included group work at the Henderson Hospital Therapeutic Community in Surrey. In 1973 I joined the staff of the Maudsley and Bethlem Royal Hospital School where I have worked both with very young children and with adolescents.

I have continued to paint since leaving Art School and in 1981 had a retrospective exhibition. I am now seconded to the Art Therapy Course at Goldsmiths' College, University of London.

———◆———

'Do you like art?'
'No, I can't do it.'

This is a characteristic answer when I ask new pupils if they enjoy art; it is evidence that they have had insufficient encouragement, have been subjected to intensive criticism or, perhaps, have been streamed towards subjects deemed 'more academic' or 'more useful'. As educationists working closely with the National Health Service, it is our job to produce a curriculum which is therapeutic and takes account of the academic, social and, especially, the emotional development of our pupils. My membership of the teaching team involves responsibility for the visual arts; it is my ideal to take artistic activity from the borderline status of a luxury only to be pursued by the 'talented', and ensure that it becomes a valued experience for each pupil, not only while they attend school, but beyond.

Consider, though, the situation of the child in the ordinary school. He or she is part of a large group fulfilling curriculum expectations and must keep up with these and consequent emotional stresses in order to survive. The school takes responsibility for education and some moral welfare, but the expectation for emotional welfare is laid at the parental door. If the teacher perceives persistent distress in a pupil, leading to an inability to concentrate, falling behind, school refusal or psychiatric illness, the responsibility for care passes to either a pastoral member of

43

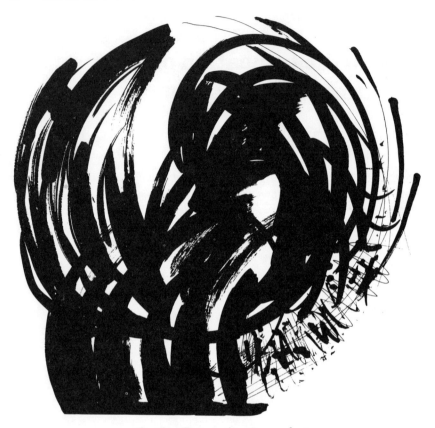

Fig. 5.1   Energy, the essence of art

staff, to the educational psychologist or another professional. The teacher may wish to play a more sympathetic role but the demands of the curriculum provide little place for such personal involvement; emotional balance in this setting is seen as enabling education to proceed, not as an aim in itself. Naturally, as a hospital school, our main priority is the emotional health of our pupils. We must accept the limitations that illness imposes on the pupils' school life, and work with whatever resources the young person possesses.

My first task with a new pupil is to make is clear that the art room belongs to all and that all the work done there is respected by me, the other pupils, teachers and the hospital staff. When I say 'work', this can mean the outpouring of emotion which is not 'art' but nevertheless matters, because it is the raw material and energy which is the essence of creation. (Fig. 5.1)

The Art Room is large and airy, sloping towards the filtered light of birchwoods. Plants, flintstones, plastic soldiers, crushed ochres and smells of graphite, paper, oil and turps give it an atmosphere inviting exploration. Into this room come young

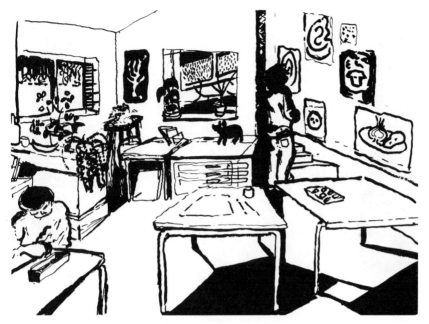

Fig. 5.2   The Art Room

people whose lives and feelings are chaotic, whose perceptions may be persecutory, needing to order their disorder and exercise their capacity to play, to experiment and to display. I look upon this room as an oasis in the school; it is informal and carefully tended. There is enough space to stretch and make life-size sculptures and group paintings. There are nooks to hide in and crannies to conceal work in until such time as confidence allows revelation. Unless a specific request is made by a pupil not to exhibit, all sorts of paintings, doodles and often pieces that a pupil does not consider worthy of display are exhibited on the walls so that there is an appreciation of the variety of expression. The overall appearance is of work 'in progress' or of growth. A 'finished product' atmosphere would nurture value judgements that are more inhibiting than liberating.

My next task is to make available different media; although there are such materials as plaster for casting, lino-cutting and silk-screening equipment on hand, I try not to overwhelm a new pupil. Materials such as paint, collage, clay, plasticine and various types of crayon have usually played some part in childhood and their familiarity can be a source of security. Observing which materials a person chooses and the way they are used gives me a first insight into the pupil.

Johnny came into my room and sat in the corner behind the plants; he began to copy carefully from a comic book and avoided attracting my attention. I could see that he wanted to get the art session over as quickly as possible and when I approached him he put his

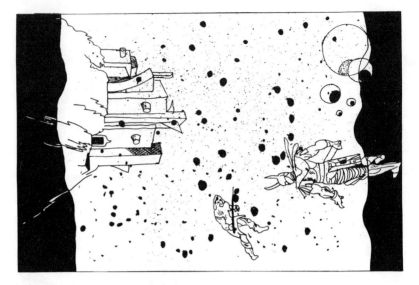

Fig. 5.3 Johnnie's painting

pictures in the drawer. For several sessions he continued in this manner, always using a pencil and always copying. Then one day he came in with another boy; neither knew what they wanted to do, but they were in a playful mood and I suggested they do a splash painting together. They started timidly and then gradually began to relax and enjoy themselves. Johnny then added blue borders to the picture and turned it into a landscape, using hero-figures that he had carefully memorised. We both discovered that he had an excellent visual memory and an ability to use colour and form dramatically. (Fig. 5.3)

I find that many depressed adolescents, school refusers and youngsters with anorexia nervosa resort to copying, tracing, or continuous pattern-making, repeating styles which have earned approval (Fig. 5.4). It is difficult for them to break away from something which has so far enabled them to scrape by without helping them to grow emotionally or artistically. These reticent creators need gentleness and patience on the part of the teacher to help them overcome their defensiveness. They need to be sure that their efforts, however small, will be received and nurtured sensitively. The effort that is made often seems regressive and a need to play is apparent; through this period expressive and kinesthetic skills are acquired, i.e. making an animal's legs strong enough to hold the body up (in clay). Finger painting or fantasising and building space cities, making and destroying and remaking are important processes which must be respected even though they may not be fully understood by either teacher or pupil. While these episodes unfold my part is similar to that of the primary school teacher, aiding but not interfering.

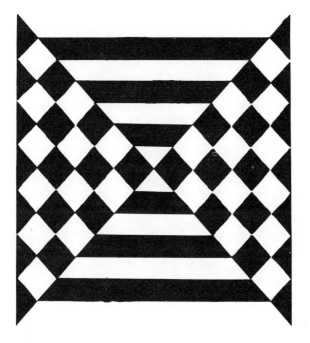

Fig. 5.4   A pattern: this does not allow the onlooker through the rigid surface

The psychotic adolescent, for example with a schizophrenic or schizoaffective disorder, may attend school either in a withdrawn or a flagrantly chaotic state. In either case he or she is often more willing to come into the Art Room than attempt personal relationships or other aspects of school. An inner dialogue while writing or painting may continue, and intervention from me is not welcomed. Several scenes may be layered on top of each other and I try to keep track of the sequence and content of these layers, so that at the end I will know that it started with three or four figures, then a boat, and that the sea gradually became stormy and the sky raged until the whole scenario became obliterated. It is not possible to understand all that is happening whilst a painting is in progress, to explain the significance of the activity or the symbols that occur, but it is necessary to have faith in the creative process.

Janie, a suicidal 15-year-old who had badly mutilated her arms and legs, participated in all lessons over-compliantly; she had always been ahead in academic work and maintained this part of her life throughout her illness even though it was obvious to us all that she cared little for either the work or herself. She was a pretty girl who wore drab, bulky clothes to cover her comeliness. During the first six weeks of admission she would come into the Art Room and curl up embryonically in the comfortable chair, not asleep, but aware of all the comings and goings, listening to the chat. On one occasion, she told me that she had not done any art since primary school – for nearly five years. It was soon after this remark that she began to bring me little drawings, done in her room on the ward: delicately pencilled hands, a pale watercoloured copy of a record-cover. All were very fragile.

One day, Janie's mood was like a black shroud, stifling her, so all-pervading that it was impossible for me not to be drawn in. I felt very strongly that this mood needed to be materialised, so I started to prepare an enormous sheet of paper, paint, but not brushes, and to pour paints on to dissolve the pristine whiteness of the paper. To my surprise (as from past experience, there is no guarantee that such an opportunity will be taken up) Janie immediately reacted; rhythmically smoothing colour over colour, filling in, texturing the space with her fingertips, until the whole surface was laden, rich and mysterious. Onto this she formed a spinning sun, its oranges and yellows harmoniously whirling with the background of brown, pinks and blacks.

When she arose, she openly showed her pleasure. She had enjoyed the sensuality of the painting, it had liberated and strengthened her. Although Janie never worked in this way again, it helped her to realise that artistic expression held unforeseen potential in her life and she started to develop her own symbolism. The previous frailty in her drawings was replaced by strong black and white paintings, experiments in charcoal, and capable hands sculpted in the pottery sessions.

Janie is a good example of a pupil who made progress by discovering new aptitudes that were genuinely her own. She could bring to the surface conflicts such as her own powerlessness against depression, finding relief and insight.

To my teaching, I have tried to bring a style which takes into account not only each pupil's personality and individual needs, but the group dynamics within the classroom. Initially, observation is important, and where the art teacher usually bustles forward with bright ideas, I hold back and discern the overall mood; this is partly because most adolescents with emotional disturbances tend to find it easier to say 'no' rather than 'yes' to other people's ideas, even if, secretly, they would like to try them out. Having said no, they then find it difficult to back down and so lose opportunities. I find it easier to have various games and themes tucked away in my head, ready.

One Friday morning six youngsters exuded lethargy from tip to toe, lolling, head on tables, eyes shut, taking ages to mix paint and asking me for pencils which were already in front of them. It was the sort of morning that can leave a teacher feeling like Sisyphus, so I asked them all to close their eyes and we did some relaxing exercises and then a guided fantasy. We imagined that we had taken a path through a forest and arrived at a hollow tree in which we found a secret passage. From there on they used their own imagination to create a picture or story. They had plenty of ideas, lethargy disappeared and a serious air of concentration took over. At the end of the session, the youngsters were amazed to find how varied were their results.

This broadly therapeutic approach does not exclude academic aims. For many children, emotional and social difficulties and low achievement go hand in hand

and helping performance helps confidence and encourages healthy development. Every year there are a few General Certificate of Education O Level exams taken in academic subjects; few are taken in Art, not because the standard of O Level is high, but because of its limited scope and expectation. The exam involves long hours, three for one paper and six for the other, and when pupils in our care have reached the stage when they are capable of dealing with the stress of this exam, they are usually well enough to be back in their own school or pursuing further education.

My own bias is towards assessment rather than examination in the Arts, so I favour the Certificate of Secondary Education (CSE), which I believe has a high standard, contrary to popular belief. The CSE exam is realistic in the way it entrusts the pupils' own teacher to mark the examination and to account to an outside examiner. The selection of at least six pieces of work over a two-year period (any form of art or craft work from jewellery to a decorated cake is exhibited) demonstrates progress and growth. The second part of the CSE is a ten-hour project, chosen from various themes. This can be divided into five two-hour periods, weekly if necessary. It is its flexibility and the emphasis on assessing art over a long period of time that makes the CSE an advance on the traditional O Level, rather than testing work as a scientific exercise with expectable answers.

When preparing for either of these exams, we work in a small group of four to eight pupils. Initially, I plan an observational project such as 'The Head', which will be explored over several weeks; one week we might look at facial expression and mood, painting and drawing very quickly on three or four sheets of paper, observing the faces around us or our own reflections. The next week we will look at skin tones, using very thin veils of paint and working slowly. A great deal of discussion goes on during these groups. Sometimes there is 'opting out' if a project seems too difficult. This 'opting out' must be dealt with carefully and on many different levels; for instance, too many options may be overwhelming the pupil and making her feel inadequate. Acknowledging difficulty in the task set may be all that is needed to reassure the youngster and get her involved again. Splitting it up into gradual steps also helps. We continue to work for the exams in the same group, but with plenty of time to do individual themes and expand on more craft skills such as plaster casting, lino-cutting and sculpture. Work done in the occupational therapy department, such as pottery, woodwork and weaving is also included in the final exam display.

The words 'control' or 'discipline' ring in every teacher's ears, and although the art class is traditionally more permissive, concentration is very important and can be easily disrupted by an argument between two disgruntled pupils. Diversionary tactics are often pursued by an unsure member of the class who does not want to reveal himself. Young people are very aware, perhaps half-consciously, just how much art does reveal. A boy may climb out of the window, wander out of the room or try to make me angry enough to send him out of the class. He may succeed in making me feel angry and frustrated, torn between the needs of the class and those of the individual, wondering whether I dare leave the class safely to coax the pupil back, or can depend on another member of staff to scoop the adolescent back into the classroom. Such behaviour can sometimes be ignored and disciplinary action or a quiet talk can take place later, but there are other times when adolescents must be dealt with on the spot.

I have described above a few adverse responses to art, one by one, but it is quite possible to have a classroom group in which all these responses take place at once. It is only through careful school management, adequate staffing levels and working with a co-operative, understanding and caring team that such problems can be minimised and an informal approach to discipline can be maintained.

Every day, staff discuss behaviour, problems and progress formally and informally. The feelings of chaos and the conflicts with which adolescents must come to terms are very strong and can powerfully affect the atmosphere of the school, just as unresolved disagreements between members of staff can affect pupils. The teaching of any subject in our school cannot be done in the same sort of isolated way that some mainstream schools expect. In order to work in a holistic way, the teacher becomes more vulnerable and personally accountable for his or her feelings and necessarily more dependent upon other members of staff. This involves a great deal of trust and the need for time to develop trust.

Twelve years ago, when I first became a member of the teaching team at Bethlem, there was little space or time given in the weekly ward round for the adolescents' artistic endeavours. It was not considered a useful contribution to the discussion. Gradually this has changed and there is now an encouraging inquisitiveness from the other members of staff about how much art can reflect the emotional dilemma of the adolescent, how it can show more than words can say. Doctors, nurses, social workers may admire an attractive work, but they are no longer beguiled by pretty pictures. They can see more clearly that the content, the ineptitude, the gauche line can contribute to understanding the myriad of reflections that can haunt or lighten the human psyche.

References and Further Reading

Berger J (1972) *Ways of Seeing*. London: BBC & Penguin Books
Bettelheim B (1976) *The Uses of Enchantment*. London: Peregrine Books
Cane F (1951, reprinted 1983) *The Artist in Each of Us*. Vermont: Art Therapy
    Publications
Dimondstein G (1974) *Exploring the Arts with Children*. London: Collier MacMillan
Ehrenzweig A (1976) *The Hidden Order of Art: A Study on the Psychology of Imagination*.
    University of California Press
Flam J D (1973) *Matisse on Art*. Oxford: Phaidon Press

Gardner H (1980) *Artful Scribbles - The Significance of Children's Drawings.* London: Jill Norman

Gulbenkian Foundation (1982) *The Arts in Schools, Principles, Practice and Provision.* Calouste Gulbenkian Foundation

Rutter M, Maughan B, Mortimer P & Ouston J (1979) *Fifteen Thousand Hours: Secondary Schools and their effects on Children.* Shepton Mallet, Somerset: Open Books

★ ★ ★

The illustrations were drawn by JM from the original works

The Adolescent Unit
Edited by Derek Steinberg
© 1986 D. Steinberg

6 Art Therapy in Practice

Diane Waller & Andrea Gilroy

Diane Waller

I studied fine art and art history at the Ruskin School of Drawing, University of Oxford and then did a two year research project on art therapy for an MA at the Royal College of Art. During this time I worked first as part time art therapist and teacher with adolescents in a psychiatric hospital, and then at the Paddington Centre for Psychotherapy where I became enthused by the ideas of Maxwell Jones and R D Laing and the concept of the therapeutic community. Between 1973 and 1977 I combined work at the Paddington Centre with introducing an art therapy option into the postgraduate Art Teacher's Certificate course at Goldsmiths' College, University of London. When this option became a postgraduate Diploma Course in 1978, the Art Therapy Unit was established and I became its Head. Most of my professional energies over the past ten years have been devoted to building up the unit and its courses, and recently to designing a higher degree course (MSc) and in being an active member of the British Association of Art Therapists, being Chairperson 1975-1981 and now Regional Officer. My research interests are in the history and development of art therapy as a profession in Britain, a topic on which I am currently completing a D Phil at the University of Sussex. From 1976-1981 I undertook training in psychotherapy. My other major interest is in the national arts of the south-east Balkans, particularly in the costumes, textiles and dance of Bulgaria and Jugoslav Macedonia. I continue to take an active part in the negotiations with the DHSS which have led to the professional recognition of art therapy within the NHS.

Andrea Gilroy

I studied fine art at the Central School of Art and Design and Canterbury College of Art. I then worked as an artist, art therapist and art teacher, training in art therapy in 1974 at Birmingham Polytechnic, and then became art therapist at Joyce Green Hospital, Kent. Since 1979 I have been lecturer to the Goldsmiths' Diploma Course in Art Therapy. Other activities include long involvement with the British Association of Art Therapists, and I have taken part in the negotiations with the Department of Health and Social Security concerning the professional recognition of art therapy. Since 1981 I have been in individual psychotherapy, and in 1983 began a D Phil at Sussex University researching the effects of art therapy on the work of artists. I try to continue my work as an artist, and in 1983 exhibited my work for the first time in many years. As to relaxation – I am a passionate gardener!

There are about five hundred art therapists currently practising in the United Kingdom. It is hardly surprising, given this small number and the fact that it is a new profession, that most members of clinical teams know little about what art therapists actually do. Art therapists often get asked questions like these:

'This person likes drawing. Would he be good at art therapy?'
'This patient wants to go to art school. Can you help him?'
'What do you think of these pictures – is this patient schizophrenic?'
'We need some decorations in the ward. Can the art therapy department help out?'
'What kind of patient would benefit from art therapy?'

In this chapter we will try to respond to these questions.

The History of Art Therapy

The term 'art therapy' was first used in Britain in 1942 by the artist Adrian Hill when he was a patient at the King Edward VII Sanatorium in Sussex. Hill had suffered from tuberculosis and found great release in being able to paint during the seemingly endless period of his convalescence. It occurred to Hill that other patients might find equal enjoyment if they could be provided with art materials and given some instruction in drawing and painting. Having persuaded the hospital authorities that this was a good idea he took materials to any patient who appeared interested, gave advice on their use and talked to the patients about the results. Hill discovered that they would often paint images resulting from war time experiences or from their illnesses. They were then able to discuss these events with Hill or a member of staff; before, they would not have been able to put into words their vague anxieties and depression. Hill therefore became, by accident, an 'art therapist', and set about convincing hospital authorities and the general public that it would be of value to have some similar facilities in other hospitals. A full account of Hill's pioneering work can be found in *'Art versus Illness'* and *'Painting out Illness'* (Hill, 1945; 1951).

Throughout the 1950s the development of art therapy was piecemeal, with art teachers, artists, psychologists and psychoanalysts working individually throughout Britain, sometimes in the NHS, sometimes privately, and meeting occasionally in working parties to try and define what this new discipline was really about and deciding who exactly would be suitable practitioners. It was when the British Association of Art Therapists (BAAT) was formed in 1964 that the role of artists and their potential for working as therapists received serious attention. One of the briefs the new BAAT Council received from the founder members was to investigate the basis of training for art therapy. Initially, art education was seen as the discipline wherein art therapy could flourish, but during 1975–76 it became clear that despite areas of common interest, art therapy and art education had become separate and distinct disciplines, the approach of the therapist and of the teacher being quite different. For example, the art therapist would place emphasis on self expression and spontaneous art work, and limit the instructional role in order to allow the patient's personal imagery to emerge.

It was during this period that the authors, as Officers of BAAT became engaged in prolonged and difficult political negotiations to have art therapy recognised as a profession in its own right, and in 1981 the Department of Health finally recognised that art therapy was a profession which warranted its own separate career and salary structure. Art therapists are now established members of multidisciplinary teams.

Background and Training of Art Therapists

Their background and training as artists gives art therapists a special understanding of art processes and symbolic communication. New entrants to the profession are usually graduates in art and design who have completed a postgraduate Diploma in Art Therapy. During their postgraduate training they become familiar with concepts in psychology and psychiatry in relation to art therapy, and with the theory and practice of psychotherapy. Having been involved in the challenge of creating images and forms themselves and finding the most appropriate means for expressing and communicating them, they are in a position to empathise with patients who are embarking on similar processes.

What art therapists do

Art therapists work in a variety of ways with a variety of people; there are as many different ways of working within the discipline of art therapy as there are within psychology or psychotherapy. To give a few examples: an art therapist may chose to work in a psychiatric outpatient clinic and work individually with patients over a long period; in a large hospital, working with groups of long-stay, chronic patients, using either a theme centred or unstructured approach; or work with families in crisis in a team using a short term, focused approach. The art therapist may work in the field of mental handicap which offers special challenges and scope, (see Stott & Males 1984).

Whatever the place of work and the theoretical approach the fundamentals of practice are similar. The art therapist provides for the patient a safe environment, free from noise and interruption, and a range of art materials which may include paint, paper, clay, water, pencils, crayons, charcoal and a variety of collage and sculpture materials. And, most importantly, the therapist provides close attention and interest throughout the session. If the art therapist is working non-directively, she will, having introduced the patient to the room and indicated the materials, wait for them to take the initiative. Many patients find this extremely hard to cope with. Being in an art room brings back all sorts of memories, especially in adults, of not being able to draw, 'being no good at art at school'. The art therapist explains that this is not important; that the expectation is not that the patient make 'good art', whatever that may be, though this is something which can take a long time for the patient to believe.

As the relationship develops the art work comes to play a crucial role in the partnership between patient and therapist. It provides a way in which the transference can be made concrete and in fact, could be described as making a kind of triangular transference: instead of relating to the therapist directly the patient may use the art work to communicate the otherwise inexpressible. In this way, the painting acts as a container for forbidden or unacknowledged feelings which can be kept and dealt with at a later stage, as well as acting as a record of the relationship and of the patient's feelings at that time. The picture may contain many time elements: the patient's childhood may be included in the same image as his present or future. Because these elements are visible and concrete, even if presented in a tentative or clumsy manner they can be shared and discussed on many levels. Like dreams they express the conscious and the unconscious, and can be unravelled or elaborated on, added to, painted over and even completely destroyed, if that is what the patient feels is important at that time.

Another way of looking at the pictures produced in art therapy is as a kind of non-verbal speech; for people with communication problems they can provide a vital outlet for expression and perhaps lead to a development in cognition. Some art therapists emphasize that the making of art is in itself beneficial and gives patients the experience of developing their latent creativity and engaging in playful activity. The self assertion needed and the sense of satisfaction achieved in making something of one's own is particularly significant for patients who have become institutionalised and lost all confidence in themselves and their abilities.

Art therapy is new in two ways. Firstly, it is officially only five years old; secondly, it offers insights and working methods which are in complete contrast to the accepted medical model in psychiatry. This has given rise to myths about art therapists and their function. Misconceptions have also arisen because of the often ambivalent attitude of the layman to art and artists. He may feel respect for and perhaps envy the skill of the artist, but be unable to comprehend the activity itself. Members of the clinical team, many of whom come from a scientific background, find themselves similarly unable to fully grasp why there is an artist in their midst. The art therapist can be regarded as a kind of shaman or witchdoctor, able 'magically' to interpret the pictures. Such a person is feared and admired. Alternatively, the art therapist can be seen as someone who encourages patients to be out of touch with reality but in touch with their unconscious. It is sometimes implied that allowing patients to paint and draw their problems and fantasy worlds can only increase their disturbance and pain. In contrast to these misperceptions is the art therapist being viewed as someone who simply gives out art materials and takes the results to the psychiatrist; such a person can easily be dispensed with.

What we do

The authors' task is to teach artists to be therapists too. Within this brief we have to function on many different and conflicting levels. We operate primarily from the position of the therapist, but in reality we are not therapists but teachers, although the students perceive us as both; an emphasis which changes as the course progresses.

Goldsmiths' students have worked for at least a year after leaving art school in an area relevant to the course. They may have had jobs as care assistants, nursing assistants, art or occupational therapy helpers, youth workers, art teachers in special schools. They are also required to have some experience of personal therapy, either individual or group. Their average age on entry for the past few years has been 30 and this year (1984) was 34. They enter a course which is highly intensive, which lasts for one year full-time or two years part-time, and which makes strenuous demands on their emotional and physical resources. The course philosophy is to link theory and practice throughout, and much of the teaching is through experiential workshops, supervision and practical placement in a wide range of institutions.

During the early part of the course, when students are attempting to readjust to their new roles, we are perceived as teachers who can give, but who more often are seen as withholding knowledge. Herein lies the first conflict, when as teachers we might wish to impart information and describe 'therapeutic techniques', whilst as therapists we know that the student has to work through the confusion, uncertainty and ambivalence which occurs at the beginning phase of the therapeutic relationship. Towards the middle of the course the dynamics change so that we are seen firmly as therapists. We also seem to become perceived as powerful parent figures, either benign or malevolent or both, whom the 'adolescent' students simultaneously need and reject. During the final phase we are perceived again as teachers, but as assessors too, with awesome powers. Disillusionment sets in: we are perceived as teachers who have pretended to be therapists. Throughout the course the student has had to tread a difficult path, taking on an 'adult' professional role in the placement, yet spending two days of the week in college where training touches on sensitive areas and provokes regression. Some of these points are illustrated in the following art therapy case study undertaken by a student (Clare) with an adolescent girl (Anna) including the point of view of the supervisors, AG and DW.

Case Study: Anna

During her first two weeks on placement in a large psychiatric hospital it was decided that Clare should work on the acute admissions ward, where more difficulty was anticipated with the younger patients with whom she might identify, than on the long-stay wards where she felt more comfortable. Almost immediately she met Anna, a 16-year-old patient who was also a newcomer to the institution. Clare's identification with Anna was immediate and very strong.

'I was shocked and surprised that such a pretty sixteen year old could be so incoherent and damaged . . . stuck in a sprawling, unfriendly institution, surrounded by chronic, mad people who seemed not to question and even to be happy with their lot. I related to her straight away.'

Anna had spent three months in another hospital and then in an assessment centre for adolescents before being admitted in a severely disturbed condition; the referral letter indicated that she had delusional ideas, loss of emotional contact, inappropriate affect and regressed behaviour including wetting and soiling. She was referred for art therapy and spent a month in open art groups before beginning to see Clare for weekly, hour long individual sessions.

Anna was one of twin girls; shortly after their birth their father had left and mother remarried when the twins were toddlers. The stepfather was said to be only interested in Anna's twin, Amanda, and the twins grew apart, Anna becoming more involved with a close friend, Louise and in time, in effect, adopted her family. Then Louise and her family moved away, leaving Anna unhappy and angry and feeling rejected by both families. At this point her mother accused the stepfather of sexually assaulting Amanda. In the following year the parental relationship worsened and stepfather left. Anna became increasingly disturbed and unmanageable, was sent to a foster home, and then to live with her stepfather. Soon after came her first admission to hospital. In the close supervision ward Anna became uncommunicative, talking and laughing to herself and spitting. She had been diagnosed acute hebephrenic schizophrenic.

In the early open art therapy groups she talked to Clare about her fear of the institution and situation in which she found herself: a fear which was most potent for Clare, who felt as lost as Anna looked. She found it hard to be the detached therapist as opposed to mother, friend, adviser and perhaps rescuer. Clare's feelings towards her college supervisors (AG and DW) were ambivalent at this stage, which was the latter half of the first term. In the supervision group (DW) Clare was defensive and put on a competent act; in individual supervision she shared her feelings of confusion and chaos. The material Clare presented was overwhelming, her notes being almost as much 'word salad' as Anna's speech. AG began to wonder where the boundaries were between herself and Anna, as well as between Anna and Clare, and after particularly difficult sessions AG too would find it hard to communicate coherently.

In an attempt to escape from her appalling situation Anna created an imaginary family. Clare felt this was reasonable in the circumstances as Anna was trying to create the good family she had never known. Anna's images were of the fantasy family, collages around the themes of home and food and pictures of cut out faces. She spoke of the 'Genie', a powerful, controlling figure who she said was responsible for her inappropriate laughter and actions, gestures and grimaces. It was the Genie who, in the pictures cut off the hair of Anna's schoolfriends, (who were envied both for their beautiful hair and their settled home lives). A month after admission Anna began drawing a 'hairy baby' and a 'hairy monkey' and linked these to the drawings of the princesses (schoolfriends) with long hair.

Clare and AG tried to make sense of Anna's art work. One approach was to examine the pictures chronologically, session by session; another was to attempt to clarify the pictures into abstract cathartic patterns, fantasy, the family and so on. Some months after Anna's admission the male art therapist mentioned that Anna often approached him in a very sexual way. Clare was away over Christmas and Anna's approaches to the male art

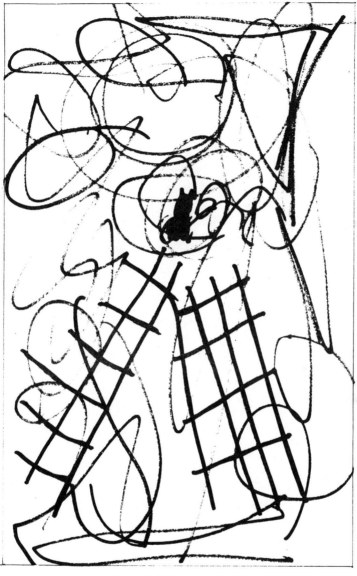

Fig. 6.1 'Kitten up a tree'

therapist became more overt. Some particularly important images appeared in art sessions: stepfather rescuing a kitten from a tree only to throw it to the ground. The picture seemed to relate to Louise's family who had 'adopted' Anna and then moved away, to her natural father who had left home, the stepfather who had also left, to Clare who had been absent over Christmas, and to the art therapist who had rejected Anna by not responding

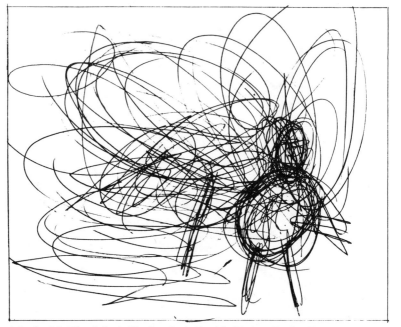

Fig. 6.2 A girl; 'No, I don't like her fat belly, it's like my Dad's. How shall I get rid of it? Anyway she's a big fat cow . . . pregnant with twin boys and twin girls'

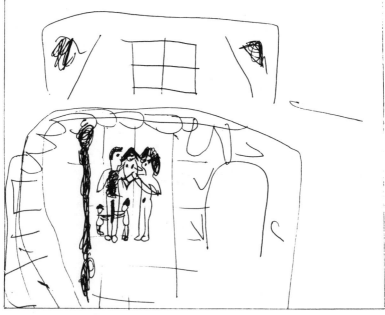

Fig. 6.3 Fantasy family 'in the kitchen'

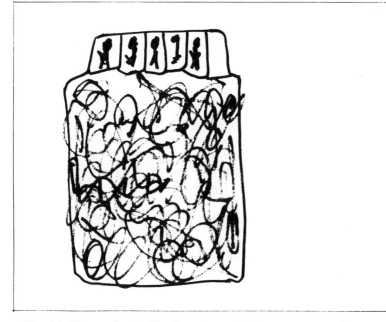

Fig. 6.4 Fantasy family: 'Family at home. Me having love and affection'

to her physical advances. The kitten could represent Anna with any of the people who had tried to care for her; after the initial rescue there was some improvement, then her hopes were dashed to the ground.

Then, with Clare, Anna drew a figure of a girl 'pregnant with twin boys and twin girls' and with a knife in the girl's belly. The stepfather visited Anna regularly and appeared to be the only member of the family interested in her well being. Clare noticed that Anna seemed more disturbed after seeing her parents, complained of feeling sick and began to lose weight. In the next few weeks she was very disturbed in art therapy sessions, working immensely hard while very distressed, and left each session physically exhausted, having alluded to a sexual relationship between herself and her stepfather. Her pictures were of a fantasy family, with Anna as a princess holding hands with characters from the Wizard of Oz or in a chauffeur-driven Rolls Royce being taken back to a happier looking house than her own home, surrounded by fictitious aunts and uncles.

In the supervision group DW felt that Clare was anxious about Anna and holding something back; she also wondered if Anna was an incest victim. In individual supervision Clare, like Anna, flooded the session with material – paintings, drawings and accounts of events. In the hospital Clare received no support for her anxieties and was told not to believe all that psychotic people say. Splits were perceived, between the supportive college and the 'bad' hospital staff, and perhaps also between AG as 'good parent' and DW as 'bad parent'. In individual supervision AG now felt like a sports coach, encouraging Clare to continue with her efforts to convey to the staff that Anna was being sexually abused by her apparently charming and concerned stepfather. Clare herself felt ambivalent about persisting; she felt Anna was being taken advantage of, yet it also seemed to be her only source of love. Then two pictures, of the fantasy family in the kitchen, and then all in bed together ('me having love and affection'), gave a clearer indication of what was happening. They both expressed the wish for closeness and unity, one being contained by the bed and the other by the kitchen boundaries. Clare felt that the kitchen picture was sexual because Anna expected this within her family and that the second indicated her distaste for her circumstances (and perhaps her wish for it to cease) as the people in bed were clearly divided, as indeed her real family were emotionally. But Anna had swopped the circumstances around, presumably because it was too painful to communicate directly. In the 'Family in the kitchen' Anna said she felt happy as she was being cuddled by both parents (she said she was the figure in the middle), but it seemed obvious that the two figures playing with the father's penis represented herself and her twin. But Anna was also between her parents, as she would be if she were having a sexual relationship with her stepfather, and in the picture the mother seems to be trying to pull her back with a rope.

A family interview was arranged, to see why Anna was disturbed after her parents' visits, and it became clear that Clare's anxieties had some basis in reality after all. She began to gain weight, socialised more and her delusions ceased. In the last session she was angry because Clare was leaving and she was not; she explained her anxieties and her behaviour coherently, e.g. wearing baggy jumpers to try to appear asexual. Clare fed back the interpretations she had made of Anna's pictures. Anna said that she was glad someone had understood her. Clare asked Anna if she would like to continue in individual therapy – art or verbal. Anna replied 'No. It's none of their business.'

The major point which this case study illustrates is that the core of Anna's problems was communicated only in art therapy. There she depicted, amongst other themes, the fantasy family and elaborated many stories about and around the characters. Perhaps this represents one of the fears mentioned earlier on in this chapter, in that Anna was encouraged to explore her fantasy world in considerable depth. But it was only through doing this that she eventually let Clare know, loud and clear, that she *was* being sexually abused.

Clare attended case reviews regularly and fed back the messages she received from Anna. The fact that for a while both Clare and Anna were not believed could be as much to do with scepticism about art therapy as with the taboo of incest (particularly with such a seemingly caring stepfather). Perhaps it is only a discipline slightly outside the central medical model, which enables patients to play – and to examine their pain and chaos whilst being contained by the image and the art therapist – that can allow material to emerge which would otherwise have remained hidden.

Conclusion

The past ten years have seen major changes and improvements in the status of art therapists in the NHS. But other employing authorities such as the social services and education need to be convinced that it would be beneficial to have an art therapist as a member of their team. We hope this task will be slightly easier now there is a structure in the NHS to use as a precedent, but we are under no illusions about the kinds of problem we sometimes face from other disciplines, particularly when art therapy is so often misunderstood. It is even the view of some artists that to mix art with therapy is to dilute or even pervert the creative process, therapy being seen as a narrow reductive process only for the sick.

What is it about art therapy that elicits such mixed feelings? To some extent we have examined them here; but perhaps art therapists have to accept that ambivalence towards them is an important and dynamic ingredient in their work, and that the sometimes uneasy partnership between art and therapy could be one of the reasons why the process is so powerful and can be startlingly successful. It is certainly a fact that art therapists, and art therapy tutors, have to be able to live with uncertainty and ambivalence, and indeed, when working with adolescents, be able to survive them and live to tell the tale.

References and Further Reading

Hill A (1945) *Art Versus Illness*. London: Allen & Unwin

Hill A (1951) *Painting Out Illness*. London: Williams & Northgate

Stott J & Males B (1984) Art therapy for people who are mentally handicapped. In Dalley, T. (ed). *Art as Therapy*. London: Tavistock

Waller D (1972) *A Personal Appraisal of Art Therapy in Britain*. MA Thesis. London: Royal College of Art.

Waller D (1984) A consideration of the similarities and differences between art teaching and art therapy. In Dalley, T. (ed) *Art as Therapy*. London: Tavistock

Waller D & James K (1984) Training in art therapy. In Dalley, T. (ed) *Art as Therapy*. London: Tavistock

Note

Information on art therapy can be obtained from the British Association of Art Therapists, 13c Northwood Road, London N6 5TL

7 Occupational Therapy with Adolescents

Diana Lockie

I trained in Edinburgh, Scotland, and held my first post at the Royal Edinburgh Hospital until Summer 1971. I then joined the staff of Netherne Hospital, Surrey and held several posts there before being appointed Head Occupational Therapist in 1975. Following the introduction of management positions for the remedial professions I became District Occupational Therapist to the East Surrey Health District until 1981, when I was appointed Director of Occupational Therapy Services to the Bethlem Royal and the Maudsley Hospitals.

I have been a Council member of the College of Occupational Therapists and have served on a number of its committees. I am currently a member of the District Occupational Therapists Committee of the College, a moderator at the Newcastle Polytechnic Occupational Therapy School and Expert Advisor in Psychiatric Rehabilitation to the World Federation of Occupational Therapists. In 1982 I undertook an assignment for the United Nations in Northern Cyprus, advising on the development of occupational therapy and rehabilitation services and providing some basic training for personnel. I am also a team member of the Health Advisory Service, and a member of the Mental Health Act Commission.

My particular professional interests include post-registration training for those working in the field of psychiatry, the evaluation of techniques, the planning and development of community based psychiatric services and the future role of the occupational therapist in relation to them.

———◆———

One of the main assets of the occupational therapist is that although she will be seen by patients as an adult figure she will not necessarily be identified so clearly as a doctor, nurse or teacher. This allows her a flexibility of approach not always achieved by members of other disciplines. It is possible, perhaps, for her to be more adaptable in finding levels of tolerance between permissiveness and limit-setting and between direct and indirect approaches. The patients may find themselves able to relate to the occupational therapist rather in the way they would to an adult friend of their family or a relative such as an aunt or uncle, which may be a close relationship without the pressure of the immediate family link.

Occupational therapy is defined as 'the treatment of physical and psychiatric conditions through specific selected activities in order to help people reach their maximum level of function and independence in all aspects of daily life' (College of Occupational Therapists, 1981). In psychiatry, occupational therapy is about the development, practice and acquisition of life skills. In other words, those predominantly practical skills and activities of daily living which enable a person to cope, even when limited to a degree by psychological difficulty, to lead as full, active and independent a life as possible.

Before the therapist begins to plan a treatment programme she will take account of current factors influencing the motivation, performance or learning ability of the adolescent. These will include clinical factors, educational background, intellectual potential, family relationships and also the therapeutic environment and resources available. She must, in addition, consider the appropriate level of function for an individual and will take account of the age, culture and social background of the patient when determining what is acceptable; in one type of culture an 11-year-old could be expected to make his bed, dress and prepare himself for school quite independently, while in another cultural group or, indeed, family quite the reverse may be the norm (Mosey 1981).

In one way occupational therapy can sometimes prove an unparalleled treatment model within a residential setting. By its very nature and organisation it is geared from the beginning to help the patient learn to cope even if quite ordinary familiar day-to-day events seem to be threatening. There is always the danger during a lengthy stay in hospital that the child may become too protected by his environment; it does, after all, provide him with many facets of life which may not have been present before: a ready made peer group, strong parental models and a structure to his day or week. Occupational therapy should always aim to help the patient towards independence by allowing scope for individual development. Sometimes hospital settings can deny opportunities to exercise decision-making or leadership skills and somehow these should be incorporated into the programme.

Occupational therapists make use both of standard techniques and practical approaches. The former, such as goal-setting, assessment, interviewing and teaching are undertaken primarily by the therapist; on the other hand, practical activities such as domestic and recreational activities and work-related skills require active participation by the patient if these are to be effective (College of Occupational Therapists 1981). Such techniques and practical skills are combined within an occupational therapy programme to produce benefit in two different directions. The therapist will employ her own techniques with the distinct aim of enhancing the self confidence, emotional maturity or self esteem of her adolescent patient. At the same time, growing self-confidence leads to improvement in undertaking the activity itself, with a corresponding development in skills. By using techniques and activities skillfully in conjunction with each other the occupational therapist can often overcome some of the initial difficulties encountered by the patient in relating to others, and so the activity becomes a catalyst.

> Jennifer is a 16-year-old girl who became depressed after her father's death; she then became excitable and unable to control her sexual behaviour. She became less able to cope at school

and could not concentrate upon her work. Following admission she arrived in the hospital school crying and would cling onto the occupational therapist's arm, often called her 'Mum', and had to be escorted to and from school. She made good use of the small groups, led by one of the occupational therapists, to talk about her father's death and other losses in the family. She started to participate in work-related activities and went on to develop responsibility for organising activities for the groups and making leaving and welcoming cards for the unit, an undertaking which reflected some of her problems and which the occupational therapist helped to put into a more constructive perspective.

Activities Used in Occupational Therapy With Adolescents

These include (i) self-care activities, (ii) career guidance and work assessment, (iii) leisure and recreational activities, (iv) self-expressive skills and (v) social skills training. Outside the hospital these skills would normally be learned and practised in a variety of different settings, for example, as part of an extra-curricular school syllabus, in clubs and more informal leisure and recreational groups, and at home with family and friends.

Self-care activities

Some individual activities such as personal hygiene and the care of clothes are usually considered to be that part of life at home which within the residential setting becomes the responsibility of the nursing staff. Activities involving beauty care and clothes are particularly important with this age group as they are often experimental media and there is considerable emphasis upon exercising choice. They allow and indeed lend themselves to the development of good peer interaction and approval. Domestic management activities embrace a broad spectrum of tasks such as menu planning, budgeting, shopping, cookery, washing and ironing and are aimed at helping the young person to prepare for living outside the hospital.

Opportunities also occur for the occupational therapist to help in introducing (or reintroducing) the use of community facilities such as shops, the post office and the bank. Sessions aim to provide guidance as well as practice; for instance, basic dietetics in menu planning in an effort to discourage a boy or girl from living solely on snacks or fast food, and in budgeting to help to plan the sensible use of money in preparation for the time when they are earning and have to be self-sufficient.

Career guidance and work assessment

Older children, particularly those of sixteen and over, may need considerable help to achieve further education, training and employability. These days there is usually an equal expectation that young people of both sexes will work on leaving school and inevitably, in a period of high unemployment, those whose education and development has been interrupted or delayed in any way will be more likely to be disadvantaged from the outset. Among some sections of society there may be greater social pressures on young men to find work and become financially independent of the family than upon unemployed girls, who may be expected to occupy at least some of their time helping with work in the house (Donovon & Oddy 1982).

The occupational therapist is in the fairly unusual position of being able to observe patients in a variety of different situations, and to be involved with them in a number of activities which make quite different demands; this helps to formulate judgements about potential areas of employment. Guidance and counselling specifically about employment issues can be helpful on an individual basis. The department can be organised to provide simulated work in which the young person can gain some experience; it must be emphasised, however, that this does not constitute training but does help to encourage such qualities as reliability, persistence and self-discipline. Work practice in other hospital departments such as the hairdressers, canteen or a clerical workshop can also provide a starting point for the adolescent to experience work routine, and allows staff to gain more knowledge about his suitability. Such aspects of assessment are particularly useful to the occupational therapist when liaising with careers officers, youth training and employment schemes organised by the Manpower Services Commission, or in some cases, day centres or sheltered employment facilities.

Leisure and recreational activities

A large number of activities fall into this category, some of which are more naturally part of the school programme, for example, swimming and other games. Occupational therapists tend to organise keep-fit and relaxation groups as opposed to more structured team games. Leisure or hobby activities may be introduced in the form of woodwork, pottery, art and other craft activities. Sometimes patients may complete individual projects; this encourages individual achievement and helps them cope with their own success, which can be a difficult experience. At other times the group may undertake a common task to encourage group involvement, sharing, helping others, making suggestions, trying out ideas and gaining reinforcement from the peer group. Often an activity such as art can be a catalyst for verbal communication. Working in a group requires tolerance of the other members yet at the same time allows for imaginative thinking and spontaneity.

Sometimes it is possible to introduce the young person to a club or group of people with similar interests well before discharge. Youth clubs or church groups may be particularly useful and form a part of the transition to normal living.

Self expressive skills

These skills include art, drama or role play and music. They are also projective techniques in that they allow an individual to project an expression of inner thoughts and conflicts into the treatment media. Sometimes they are used to aid peer and staff interaction, and as they have relatively less structure encourage the adolescent to take responsibility for himself and his actions. If skillfully used by experienced staff these activities can be useful adjuncts to psychotherapy, particularly in the earlier stages of treatment before the full extent of the patient's strengths and weaknesses are known. The adult feeds in new challenges and helps the adolescent to discover the limits of materials and situations (Bell 1977).

Social skills training

Here attention is directed to effective communication skills which can be practised in a variety of settings within the hospital and outside. Role play and interaction in small groups are important facets of the learning process here. It can be a focus both for defining problem areas and managing them.

> John was a sixteen year old who on admission acted in a bizarre way and held beliefs that his father, who had died the previous year, had been poisoned because he was good at his factory job. He was diagnosed as having a personality disorder with marked mood swings. The aims of occupational therapy with John were:
> (a) To develop an individual relationship in which he could learn to trust an adult and share some of his practical and emotional problems in preparing to go out to work, while continuing to live at home with his mother and brother and coping with the feelings in the home.
> (b) To encourage the family to support John in those areas where he could succeed, such as at college; pursuing his interest and talent in music; and in finding acceptable limits for his handling of money, which was problematic.
> (c) To encourage him to be more in touch with reality rather than allowing him to indulge excessively in fantasy, particularly in regard to sexual difficulties with girls.
> (d) To help him to improve his appearance and hygiene.
> The occupational therapist worked with John on an individual basis and in small groups using a variety of techniques. She also became involved in seeing John with his family to help them all to modify attitudes and accept change.
> His programme included self care activities, budgeting, work practice, social skills training and joining a youth club outside the hospital where he could develop realistic relationships with boys and girls of his own age. Participation in these activities provided him with opportunities he needed to achieve independence, while at the same time he was able to find and test methods of solving some of his emotional difficulties in establishing his self-image and self-esteem and relating to family and friends. He was discharged to attend a part-time basic skills course, and then entered full-time employment as a swimming pool attendant; and he now has a girlfriend.

The Occupational Therapist and Other Disciplines

The experienced occupational therapist should be able to provide a useful and unique perspective about the patient and this can act as a pivot in focusing the attention of the multidisciplinary team upon realistic rehabilitative goals for an individual. Her concentration upon this aspect of treatment together with her experience of demands in the community should enable the therapist to speak with authority on the question of the potential independence of the patient in another setting.

In adolescent psychiatry, in particular, other team members may be confused by the apparent overlap between the roles of the occupational therapist and the educationalists. Superficially the same activities may be used though their intrinsic purpose may be quite different, and it is important that these two groups of staff should be clear about their objectives. The goal of therapists and educators working in a school should be to create an atmosphere in which various approaches can develop which complement rather than oppose each other (Ottenbacher 1982).

Often teamwork with adolescent patients involves different disciplines working together with patients simultaneously, requiring agreement about who will take greater responsibility for which particular aspect of a comprehensive treatment programme. Individual members of staff may have a flair for a particular approach; a common example is in counselling. It may be more appropriate to select the person most skilled to undertake this than define the responsibility on the basis of professional background. Such overlapping of roles can usually occur only in a climate where staff feel secure and unthreatened by the skills and knowledge of others, and are free to contribute equally within the team and suggest changes or introduce new concepts. When there is disagreement as opposed to conflict the team is in a healthy state, and one in which learning can occur. Consistent conflict, however, can be destructive and disabling to a team, and this will adversely affect patient care.

Training and the Future

The College of Occupational Therapists has recently reviewed its basic training syllabus, and a gradual conversion to the new model syllabus 81 will be completed by 1985. The Way Ahead, (College of Occupational Therapists 1981) states 'A developing special interest within the profession is children who are undergoing treatment or who are at risk' and the report acknowledges that health care services for these children is one of the further priority areas planned by the DHSS. However, it would be idealistic to assume that over the next decade there will be a substantial increase in the numbers of occupational therapists practising in the field of child and adolescent psychiatry. It is hoped that those small numbers of trained people who choose this field will be able to gain experience in the speciality at the outset of their careers. All too often, at present, the specialist aspects of psychiatry have to be provided in the first career post; this limits the contribution of any newly qualified member of the profession during the first six to twelve months, and it would be preferable for the period to be considered a post-registration training year in some specialities. The small number of occupational therapists who specialise in child or adolescent psychiatry, however, will at present have limited career development prospects.

Psychiatric and other services for children and adolescents have developed and undergone considerable change in recent years. It is important that the occupational therapist, concerned as she is with the impact of adolescence upon the individual and such transitions as that from the organised structure of schooldays to the independence and choice imposed by adult life, should herself be adaptable enough to broaden her sphere of involvement to include, for example, working in the community as well as in the hospital setting.

References and Further Reading

Bell V (1977) Occupational therapy with young disturbed adolescents. *British Journal of Occupational Therapy*, **5**, 116-117

British Association of Occupational Therapists (1981) *The Way Ahead*. Report of a Working Party. London: British Association of Occupational Therapists

Bumphrey E E (1984) Occupational therapy in a health district - an overview. *Health Trends*, **16**, 86-90

College of Occupational Therapists (1981) *Diploma Course 1981*. London: College of Occupational Therapists

Donovan A & Oddy M (1982) Psychological aspects of unemployment: an investigation into the emotional and social adjustment of school leavers. *Journal of Adolescence*, **5**, 15-30

Mosey A C (1981) *Occupational Therapy Configuration of a Profession*. New York: Raven Press

Ottenbacher K (1982) Occupational therapy and special education: some issues and concerns related to Public Law 94-142. *American Journal of Occupational Therapy*, **36**, 81-84

Wilmer H A (1981) Defining and understanding the therapeutic community. *Hospital Community Psychiatry*, **32**, 95-99

Wilson M (1984) Occupational Therapy in Short-Term Psychiatry. Edinburgh: Churchill Livingstone

The Adolescent Unit
Edited by Derek Steinberg
© 1986 D. Steinberg

8 Creative Therapy

Barry Wynn

It is creative apperception more than anything else that makes the individual feel that life is worth living.

D W Winnicott   Playing and Reality

I left school with no O Levels and one RSA Certificate in English to call an examination. I was being prepared for factories, part of the social fodder of secondary school education; implicit in this was the theme that for us the lower rungs of the social ladder were quite enough. This idea was greatly helped by my mother whose range of stock phrases was very wide; one of them being 'Now Bar, get a good job in a factory won't you?'.

Unable to tolerate the atmosphere of the London suburbs, I left home at 16, went to Cornwall and generally led a fairly 'beatnik' existence for a few years. I had had three poems accepted by a local newspaper so I decided to become a writer. I'm still trying. At 21 I went to night school having become tired of dead end jobs and obtained three O Levels and then more O and A Levels during the next three years. At about twenty-five I went to a Teacher's Training College believing naively that this was comparable to a polytechnic or university. Some disillusionment followed but then I went to work in a clinic in Devon and found the therapeutic work there highly stimulating and satisfying. Writing was a lonely occupation, often arduous and unpaid; therapy involved contact with others on a more profound and intimate level. It provided a window into other people's lives that I needed in order to understand my own.

I returned to London from Devon and began to train in the creative therapies in drama therapy, art therapy, psychodrama and now as a psychotherapist with the Minster Centre for Humanistic and Analytic Psychotherapy. I still write, draw and paint, and the surge of creativity still overtakes me. The opening of a creative act leads from one daydream to another; imagination takes over and a flow of fantasy and productivity can emerge. Sometimes in writing a poem I can almost allow the words to come from another source, an unconscious part of me that 'knows' the form I want to take. Later, in revising the poem I often come back to the original words that I used, realising that the succinctness of phrase and the breadth of meaning is all there in the original version.

Creative Action

This spontaneous 'letting go' is well recorded in writing on the nature of creativity. Ehrenzweig has called the process 'differentiation' or 'unconscious scanning' and suggests that it is essential to all creative works as it entails a letting go that produces an oceanic image. The image is actually unconscious but has a structural sense of its own. This 'hidden order' will take over if the artist or creator will allow it and the fear of chaos and disintegration does not become too strong. It is something that I believe we all possess, but allowing it to come to the surface can be difficult. Koestler feels that creation comes from regressing to this unconscious place and uses the work of psychotherapy as an example. He suggests that psychotherapy aims at undoing 'faulty integrations' by taking the client back to an earlier period, so that the experience will be integrated in the psyche and therefore more controllable. Treatments such as neurosurgery and electroshock therapy perhaps release the brain's older centres from 'cortical restraints'. So psychotherapists, in a gentler way, try to help the client understand unconscious and infantile feelings and so regenerate into 'a more or less newborn person' (Koestler 1964).

This process he describes generally in terms of analogy: 'reculer pour mieux sauter' – run back to get a better jump – and is fundamental to creative and therapeutic experiences. What therapists attempt to do the unconscious can also accomplish spontaneously and naturally. It is the awakening of this spontaneity that creative therapy attempts to tap using both the creative instinct and therapeutic skill. J L Moreno, the founder of psychodrama, believed that spontaneity is an undeveloped factor in human beings and that spontaneity training can improve our responses to unexpected situations and enable us to live more creatively.

According to Moreno, spontaneity is the source of creative or dramatic skill; as children we 'play out' later life and these enacted scenes are conceived as dreams or ideals. It is this process that helps the personality mature and hence a psychodrama director would give the clients roles that they did not experience in their lives. This experiencing of so far unlived roles will then enable the personality to develop and integrate more fully (Moreno 1977). Psychodrama is a way of helping people act more spontaneously and creatively; it is psychotherapy in action. The phrase 'reculer pour mieux sauter' is particularly apt for this type of therapy: painful or difficult areas of a person's life are re-enacted and new ways of coping are dramatised. The effect can be one of profound change.

Using creative therapy with adolescents can be extremely difficult as it involves reaching back and playing in a way that young people are trying very hard to distance themselves from in order to be 'grown up'. It encroaches on that uncertain borderland between adulthood and childhood. It is taking them back so they can try a better jump almost before the jump has been taken. At this stage in human development there is uncertainty about the future, a longing for honesty and reason in what seems a disordered and chaotic world – both the inner world and the outer reality that the adolescent perceives. Confusion over roles, sexuality and a place in the world are all inherent in a young person's actions, as is the often contemptuous rejection of the values of adults.

The negative perceptions of the adolescent need to be countered by positive regard and a firm belief by the adult therapist in the value of the work he is doing. Many times have I had the feeling 'What's the point, no-one wants to know, they're not interested, it's all boring'. If this adolescent feeling then feeds into my own negative feelings and doubts, the result is a stalemate or blocking that becomes thoroughly self-defeating. For example, I want to start a game: various responses could be, 'No, I don't want to', 'Load of shit', 'I'm going to do something else', 'We want to talk' and so on. Perhaps one or two people will show interest and some enthusiasm for joining in, and if I then start the game with these few plus another member of staff, others may become involved. This involvement sparks an interest in an onlooker and in someone else who was bored and who may also join in; it then becomes possible to begin working cooperatively. Ideas that don't work are common; people wander off part-way through a game, one or more saboteurs break up a session, something that works one time may fail at another. Persistence, humour and a resistance to initial disappointment are needed in great supply. The rewards may never be visibly substantial but they are there; the therapist is not owed a reward from the young people he is working with and, in turn, adolescents find it difficult to give positive or encouraging responses. They can do this, but it may be very difficult to discern exactly what affection is there especially if it comes in the form of a punch or a swearword. In a world where it is suddenly difficult to trust anything, including the body's own feelings, the expression of caring for someone may take peculiar forms. It is important to recognise that this may happen; it is not worth patronising or making up to the young person concerned. Expecting too much may be a function of the therapist's own needs and there should, as with all similar work of a difficult nature, be supervision and support from colleagues and other disciplines.

Creative therapy as a profession is just beginning to expand, and who should supervise this type of therapy is an open question. Are psychiatrists or psychologists necessarily qualified to supervise what is usually a different type of practice from their own? Certainly there needs to be a support system and interstaff supervision. As this specialism grows so will the need for qualified supervision; at present, this need is largely unmet, although the British Association of Dramatherapy has recently inaugurated a supervisor's course. One hopes that as the profession expands this area may be given more serious thought.

The Beginnings of a Group

For the creative therapist acceptance by other staff is essential. Other members of the team are needed to provide adult models and to guide and encourage reluctant members of the group to participate. I find they can also help me if I give an unclear instruction by asking for clarification, which is something that the adolescent group might not do. Preliminary discussion is needed with other staff about the requirements of participation, their own willingness to attend and the time and place available.

On one occasion, I took some lesson time within the school when all the young people in the unit would be there. Some of the staff of the school agreed to attend the group. While I gave the instructions and directed, they would participate in the activities. We used to meet in a hut that was unoccupied in the late morning. The group would just be called 'Barry's group'. This was to avoid the connotations of calling it dramatherapy or psychodrama and promoting expectations of doing drama and nothing else. Sometimes we would start on time, occasionally there was a feeling of reluctance either in myself, amongst the adolescents or from other members of staff. This is understandable in that there was a change in power relation from my position as teacher to that of creative therapist; creative groupwork can be challenging and unpredictable, consequently there is some resistance to working in this way; some of the themes explored can be upsetting for adults and children alike and there could be a sense of being exposed and revealing too much as a professional. We invited other professions to participate and a nurse and the unit's occupational therapist would attend regularly.

Although employed as a teacher in the unit's school, I also functioned as a counsellor and groupworker. The role change to group leader did not seem to affect the young people who participated and did not create a role conflict within me, which I felt reflected the unit with its diverse multidisciplinary input. This may have been felt by other staff, however, which is an issue I shall return to later in the chapter.

A Typical Session

Two or three people are assembled including myself. I worry where the others have gone since it is only a short walk from the unit to the hut where we work. Old feelings of anxiety and self-doubt form in my mind and I allow myself to drift over what could go wrong for a few seconds, then dismiss these feelings by concentrating on the practical steps of the session. Starting and being involved in creative therapy is very much thinking on your feet; if something unexpected happens the group may go a very different way. I run over techniques, ideas, check my notes. A few more drift in, two, then three girls who make a huddle near the fire and become involved in giggling and whispering, seemingly engrossed in each other. Christopher, an immature 17-year-old, runs noisily round the room, throwing cushions and poking the girls; a member of staff admonishes him. I choose to hold back, not wanting to begin in a punitive way. There are enough people to start now so I raise my voice, suggesting we begin. This is generally ignored although one boy dodges round me touching me quickly and nervously as if I am about to disappear, saying 'What're we gonna do this week Barry? Eh? What're we gonna do?'. I answer inscrutably 'Wait and see'.

I raise my voice again, not shouting but carrying the voice and suggest that it is time to start. One or two children respond; so do the staff. I get them into a rough circle and ask them to shake out and loosen up, first one hand and then the other, making it as floppy as possible. Then one foot, making it as loose on the ankle as possible, then the other, then both together – a joke. Then shake out all the arms, shoulders and whole body and then close eyes. I am reassuring about this saying 'Close your eyes if you feel you can; some people may find it difficult to do this. Move around carefully among the group until you meet someone, open your eyes, take their arm and massage it up and down with both hands from wrist to shoulder; change sides; and then change over so your partner does the same back to you'. So far about half the group seem partly interested.

Now I want to involve as many people as possible so I suggest a game. A kind of 'it' where one person is 'it' and chases the others. To escape being caught one person has to be lifted off the floor by another, then neither can be caught. Sneering disbelief from a section of the audience. Some of the staff start, and a few of the more adventurous adolescents. It's enjoyable, and a few more join in. A riot. Shouts, screams, lots of laughter, now I've made two people 'it' instead of one so that the action is faster. A lot of the group are involved now, there's much activity and spontaneous contact. I like the success but don't want it to go on for too long in case the energy drops and it becomes difficult to move on from here. People become tired, rest a bit, panting, look to me. I leave it a few moments longer so that the exhuberant energy subsides, then suggest that each person takes a partner, the same as in the warm-up or someone different, find a space in the room and sit down there. Now I ask them to share with each other what they feel are issues for them in the unit; one starts while the other listens, then change round and compare ideas. More people join in than before, quite a lot of conversations start, some on the instructions, others about football or unit gossip (an issue in itself). I have less than an hour; do I want them to go into fours and share what they have said in a smaller group? I decide against this and leave them talking for a few minutes. When I notice that some people have stopped I move the session on by suggesting that I shall use a chair to represent issues that were discussed and invite people, still with their partners, to say what were the issues they talked about. A pause. Then one person, perhaps a member of staff, says 'Friendship was an issue that we talked about.' I try to clarify:

'You mean making friends? Losing them? Or people being friendly to each other?'

'Making friends mainly, whether people want to be friends or have friends at all!'

I put out a chair in the central space as most of the group are around the perimeter of the room; this chair represents friendship. There is another pause. A member of staff encourages Leroy to say what they were talking about. He says shortly 'Getting out of this place.' I reflect back:

'Getting out of this place, wanting to leave as soon as possible, escaping from here. Leaving – shall we call it that?'

General assent, and so I put out a chair that represents leaving. This process continues until we have five chairs around the room including the two already mentioned. The other subjects covered are tea money, families, gossip, and one other chair. I introduced the gossip chair as I said that I felt this was an issue in the group, and it was something I felt should not be left out. I say about the sixth chair, and about the theme we will follow:

'Okay, these chairs represent various issues that are around in the unit. This last chair that I'm holding represents "how can we change it?" How are things going to change, be better? Some kind of resolutions can be suggested in this chair unless we get stuck in an unsolveable argument. What I'd like people to do is to sit in any chair and say what comes up for them, what they feel like saying about the issue that chair represents. And then let's use this chair, which I'll put in the middle, as a means of changing; can it be changed?'

There is a pause as people take in what I have said. No one says he does not understand what I mean. The silence is tense, expectant. One of the girls picks up on a rumour that has been going round that a boy was in one of the girl's rooms, then, giggling, says she doesn't really want to mention it. She is persuaded to sit in the chair and does so, reluctantly. Different adolescents are at different stages of maturity; some dismiss all this as crap, some giggle or act out, one or two girls encourage Julie to say more. She does so and they pick up the theme seriously and with concern. The real work of the group has started.

One boy is repeating his name in a corner of the room, going from high to low pitch; an 18-year-old suddenly runs out of the room. I ignore this but another member of staff reacts and follows him out to try to persuade him to come back. Interruptions like these are frequent and need to be taken as they occur without too much anxiety from the group leader. As the group becomes educated in the methods that are being used some will come to value the experience and work with the techniques; others will find it too threatening and there will be disruption, especially in the initial stages of the session. But when key issues are out in the open intense concentration replaces the earlier chaos. In this electric atmosphere the therapist observes the real purpose and satisfaction of this work. This group continued with active discussion and looked at painful and difficult issues. The technique of using chairs to represent issues or relevant other people is widely used in Gestalt therapy and psychodrama: the empty chair. It also helps to prevent a group from becoming too static; if someone has to change chairs to express ideas this movement is a mini warm-up in itself.

Techniques

Warm-up is physical activity to relax the group and increase energy and communication. It can also be a preparation for the work ahead and may include some of the themes of the session. *Games* are a secondary phase of warm-up and encourage cooperation, contact and a stepping back to childhood excitement and the immediacy of experience. If people are seated I will often start the warm-up from the floor or chairs, using what is being sat upon as part of the process. Occasionally, I have spent whole sessions playing games – to great effect.

The empty chair can be used to represent an absent person whom the protagonist can address. A dialogue can be developed from this by *role reversal*, for example an adolescent playing herself and her mother in an argument.

Doubling is widely used in dramatherapy. The double imitates the posture of someone else, expressing his unspoken thoughts and feelings as they seem to be. These things will need to be openly stated to complete the process; the role of the double (which I may take if someone seems particularly stuck) is to aid this expression.

Sculpting means making a sculpture out of people in the group to express feelings and relationships or to clarify underlying dynamic processes. It may be used to look at group structure and relationships, to consider aspects of authority; to illustrate an individual's feelings about himself, or to demonstrate relationships in a family. For example, if someone says 'Dad's out at the pub every night, my brother and sister are always out and Mum's always watching TV', then members of the group can be used to illustrate the positions, postures and relative positions of the family members in a sculpt; each person then says how it feels to be in that position. They can be doubled by the person who made the sculpture. Sometimes the visual impact may seem enough in itself and discussion may follow on the way it looked. Sculpts can also be changed to an ideal situation or to more comfortable relationships between its parts.

Mirroring is a psychodramatic technique which, by using other group members, shows a person his behaviour as if in a mirror. The leader may ask a person to sit out of a situation he is enacting and in which he is obviously stuck; someone else takes that person's role and the scene is played again so that the original actor may see how it looks from the outside. The individual becomes an audience to his own actions. The director could then ask other people to replay the scene in a different way, to show how they would change this situation: the original person is then asked to go back into the same scene and change it as he would like it to be. Thus adolescents are able to observe the effect of often thoughtless actions and become aware how these actions may effect others.

Mirroring illustrates how a person behaves and enables him to observe this behaviour and evaluate its effectiveness, as well as practising change in a safe, uncritical way.

Role reversal is perhaps one of the most important therapeutic tools that psychodrama has given therapists and a remarkably effective way of seeing another's point of view. If the empty chair is being used, for example, and a son is talking to his mother, he can change roles and become his mother and respond as she would, then change back and respond, and so on. Whan an auxiliary (another member of staff), playing an important other person, is asked a question that he has difficulty in answering (eg. 'Why didn't you give me enough love as a child?'), the protagonist can then reverse roles with the auxiliary and answer that question as the parent, gaining some idea of the parent's way of thinking or a particular way of behaving. Role reversal provides a stimulus to the imagination; in taking on the other person's role scattered information may be assembled and finally understood.

Individual Work

Undertaking counselling or psychotherapy with adolescents is notoriously difficult, especially when using traditional approaches in which the therapist is an arbitrary, non-judgmental figure who does not share any experience or emotion of his own, but sits and says almost nothing. This approach, in my view, is an unsatisfactory one, as all the power resides in the therapist and none in the client – not the best of models for young people who are struggling with their own power relationships with parents, society and themselves.

Szasz (1979) describes psychotherapy as a form of personal influence in which one person, the therapist, is supposed to exert a considerable therapeutic influence on another person, the client. But then in countless *other* situations people influence each other and, as Sasz puts it, '. . . who is to say whether or when such interactions are helpful or harmful and to whom?'. This raises the questions whether, how or why psychotherapy is effective. I would attempt a limited answer by surmising that provided both the identified therapist and the identified client feel some empathy between each other then the interaction can be positive. With young people there is a need to be relaxed and positive as well as being prepared to share relevant personal material in a professional way. I try to encourage a sense of relaxation by making a cup of tea or coffee before a session and being active with my own things as well as responding to the young person present. I find this puts the child or adolescent more at ease. We work in a room that has paints, clay and writing materials available and we may paint or draw simultaneously; this can promote empathy in the act of doing and enables me to ask casual and indirect questions as opposed to direct questions that may lead to long, fruitless silences.

Denise was a girl who had great difficulty making relationships with men due to the brutality of her father towards her. I was told that she would be forthcoming at first but then clam up to the point where she would not appear for sessions and no further headway could be made. We began each session by making tea or coffee and having a general conversation about her school work, jobs and what she has been doing that week. We then moved to the art room and used paint and, on one occasion, clay. I encouraged her to draw a diagram of family relationships by making one of my own and discussing it with her. I did not make too many interpretations about her work but observed what she was doing and asked questions so that a picture gradually emerged. She had strong incestual fears about her father, a theme that was graphically suggested in symbolising her mother as a cushion between herself as a teddy bear and her father as a sharp dagger. My understanding of the family dynamics was helped by seeing a video of a family therapy session with Denise, father and mother, and this gave me further clues to follow, such as asking Denise where each member of the family would sit if they were all watching television, and then to portray it in paint.

We worked in this way for an hour once a week for three months, supplemented by the adolescent group that she also attended. She came along quite regularly, invariably apologising if, for some reason, she was unable to attend. In our final session she confirmed that when seeing someone individually before she had quickly become bored and avoided going. This had been 'different' somehow and she had enjoyed our sessions, a feeling that was reciprocated.

Individually or in groups, adolescents need to be treated with respect and as thinking people. This does not mean never getting annoyed or not being firm, but being as honest as possible and prepared to share something of one's own life in order to reflect their own.

Working with Staff

Creative work can be as inhibiting for staff as it is for adolescents; there may be feelings of jealousy ('Is he more creative than I?'), or memories of personal failures at school in art or drama ('I can't draw; I can't act!'). These feelings need to be understood by the therapist. Resistance can also arise from staff if the work undertaken touches upon unresolved areas of difficulty for them, or if someone in the group becomes particularly upset. Ideally, the other staff in a dramatherapy or psychodrama group (who are called auxiliaries) will have had some experience of these techniques before; often this is not the case, however, and the group leader needs to be reassuring and convincing about his work.

Initially, all those involved with the unit should be informed that the group will take place, when, and where and the type of group, and that they are welcome to attend. Written invitations may be a positive encouragement for staff who might feel excluded. One way of involving and teaching colleagues is to run a workshop to demonstrate techniques.

Conclusions

One problem of which the creative therapist has to be aware is that his work, as a therapeutic activity, may overlap the more formal counselling or psychotherapy being undertaken by one of his colleagues. It is important to use the groups and meetings where work with the children is planned, discussed and reviewed.

The creative therapist has other difficulties, too. There is a culturally entrenched idea that 'creators' are likely to be feckless, immoral people whose work, while sometimes given almost mythical status, is also not believed to be scientific, sensible, practical or even wholly sane. Freud admitted he had little time for cultural pursuits and saw creativity as an extreme of egoistic narcissism serving as an outlet for manic-depressive or neurotic tendencies (eg. Freud 1922). Jung took creativity more seriously and used painting and drawing when seeing his clients (Jung 1954). Interestingly, however, Freud used art in the form of myth to illustrate one of his most famous concepts, Oedipal conflict. From a sense of dissatisfaction with classical analysis, Moreno (1977) began to use drama in Vienna in the 1920s and started a group called the *Living Newspaper* in which news stories were enacted on a stage. Milner (1950), Winnicott (1971) and others have added to the development of creativity as an adjunct to psychodynamic understanding and therapy, but dissidence to the strictures of psychoanalysis and to the cultural stereotype of artistic activity continues to this day, and the various arguments are represented also in the proliferation of the literature of Humanistic Psychology and the so-called 'growth' group. Prevalent in this movement is a sense of trying to bring order to chaos, within the individual as well as without. The act of creation helps bring some order to chaos, and the joy it can provide is often without measure.

References and Further Reading

Blatner H (1973) *Acting In.* Berlin: Springer
Ehrenzweig A (1967) *The Hidden Order of Art.* London: Weidenfeld Nicolson
Freud S (1922) *Introductory Lectures on Psychoanalysis.* London: Routledge & Kegan Paul
Jennings S (1973) *Remedial Drama.* London: Pitman
Jennings S (1975) *Creative Therapy.* London: Pitman
Jung C G (1954) *The Practice of Psychotherapy.* London: Routledge & Kegan Paul
Koestler A (1964) *The Act of Creation.* London: Macmillan
Langley D and Langley G (1983) *Dramatherapy and Psychiatry.* London: Croom Helm
Milner M (1950) *On not being able to Paint.* London: Heinemann Educational Books
Moreno J (1977) *Psychodrama, Volume 1.* New York: Beacon Press
Starr A (1967) *Psychodrama: Rehearsal for Living.* Chicago: Nelson Hall
Szasz T (1979) *The Myth of Psychotherapy.* New York: Doubleday

Dramatherapy is the Journal of the British Association of Dramatherapy, and is available from the Editor, 7 Hatfield Road, St Albans, Herts

The Adolescent Unit
Edited by Derek Steinberg
© 1986 D. Steinberg

9 Family Therapy and an Adolescent Inpatient Unit

Christopher Dare

I qualified in medicine and psychology at the University of Cambridge. After clinical qualification and general medical experience at Guy's Hospital, I trained as a psychiatrist at the Maudsley Hospital and then moved to the Tavistock Clinic to train in child psychiatry, where I completed my training as a psychoanalyst. At the Tavistock Clinic I became involved in the beginnings of family therapy. Since being appointed to the staff of the Maudsley Hospital I have been involved in the development of family therapy there. I have maintained a practice as a psychoanalytic psychotherapist.

———◆———

This chapter is written as an outcome of leading regular family therapy seminars in the Adolescent Unit at Bethlem Royal Hospital, which began when whole-family meetings began to play an increasing part in the treatment plans of the unit. The seminars consist of a weekly hour-long multidisciplinary meeting, the major participants being the staff social workers, registrars and senior registrars, and those members of the senior nursing staff involved in important family contacts, occasionally joined by outside workers involved with one or other of the young people on the ward. Students in the various disciplines also attend.

Initially, the title of the meeting varied. Then, some years back, following collaboration with the unit's Director, Derek Steinberg, and other members of the Children's and Adolescents' Department on the subject of consultation (see Yule *et al*, 1983), we decided that the most sensible designation for this weekly family therapy event was *consultation*. As family therapy consultant I do not have managerial responsibility for ward functioning or for the clinical conduct of those attending, and the seminar has been conducted with careful concern for the established supervising executive authority. This feature has structured the nature of my input. Negotiations within the unit as to which professionals should attend has been important; while most of the unit's workers are likely to believe in the relevance of family therapy discussions, attendance at the seminars has been restricted to those active with the families of youngsters who were the unit's responsibility. Another influence on the nature of the consultative work described in this chapter has been my work with residential homes for young people in the London Borough of Southwark, and who represent another group of children and adolescents living outside their families.

General Principles of Family Therapy

General systems theory (Gorell-Barnes 1984) is concerned with the rules that govern the relationship between the complicated elements that make up biological systems within an overall ecology, and is the most influential theoretical basis for family therapy. Systems theory suggests that the way to understand how a family works and discern the rules governing its behaviour is to see the whole family in interaction, rather than to gain detailed knowledge of individual functioning away from the family. A family therapist is much more concerned with viewing the family as a whole than seeking cause of disorder in individual functioning; a symptom of an individual is ascribed to properties of the family rather than assigned to an individual. Correspondingly, family therapy is directed towards enabling the whole family to be involved in finding resources to change the functioning of the family as a unit. A change is sought in the initial perception of presenting problems away from seeing it solely as the 'property' of individual members, by enabling the family to find different ways of carrying out their joint tasks. This is achieved by using the following four groups of techniques.

1 Engagement and joining

The family therapist is responsible for covening meetings which contain as many family members as possible. In general, for beginners, and at the beginning of all family therapies, meetings containing less than the whole household should not be accepted as useful. The authority of a professional agency for the mode of conduct of its job is highest in the early stages of contact, and if a meeting of the whole household is made an important condition of effective work at this stage many problems in convening whole-family gatherings will be diminished. The therapist must make sure that each family member feels his point of view and presence are respected and welcomed; this is done by ensuring that each family member has some moments of interaction with the therapist to indicate that they are expected to express opinions about the nature of the problem, its causes, and how the family might go about doing something about it. Each family or household member should believe that the therapist expects them all to gain some advantage from family therapy, and this is particularly important for adolescent siblings of a nominated adolescent patient.

2 Defining the problem

The family therapist should seek to negotiate a consensually acceptable definition of the problem. Usually, important family members nominate the problem as the prerequisite of one member; the family therapist should respect this but should try to translate the problem assigned to one family member as having implications for the interactions between that member and others. For example, if a youngster is depressed and the parents say to the therapist 'our problem is that our son is deeply miserable' then the therapist would try to explore the effects of that misery on the other family members and would seek acceptance of a definition of the problem in terms of those effects. 'You have come to see me, I see, because you are all desperately upset and puzzled by your son's misery. Can you help me more by telling me how this extreme misery on the part of your son affects each of you individually? I expect that because you are all rather different people you have different responses and perhaps hear about different aspects of his misery. Could you tell me more about that?' It is not necessarily sensible for the therapist to inform the family that he is trying to stop the problem being seen as belonging to the patient, but to carry the family along with him by the process of consensual re-definition. Each family member should be left with a memory which enables him to state the reason for attendance; that reason should be meaningful and sensible to him.

3 The development of the family therapist's understanding of the problem

The family therapist will need to evolve an understanding of the way the family works in relation to the presenting problems, noting the following general points.

(i) It is crass for a family therapist to believe that all families function in the same way and to be unaware of class and ethnic influences on the conduct of families within their community of clinical responsibility. Expectations about adolescent freedom, for example, vary enormously in different cultural groups. Sociocultural and historical influences are probably the most important factors in determining how particular families conduct family business.

(ii) Within the sociocultural framework, intergenerationally transmitted factors also determine the way a family expects family life to be conducted; the way roles are assigned to the different parents and the balance of autonomy and control within the general family activity pattern; the sources and mode of communication of identity expectations of adolescence, and so on. How parents expect themselves and their children to behave will be affected in detail by the reality and the fantasy about their family of origin experiences. At some stage in the course of any persisting family therapy it will usually become sensible to draw up a family tree and to enquire as to the forebears of the family to facilitate the therapist's understanding of these intergenerational processes. The timing of this must be flexible.

(iii) The most important initial feature of a family diagnosis should involve assessment of the features of life cycle location of the family members; each person in the family should be seen as undergoing, in the course of his own life a series of developmental phases (Erikson, 1959). Passage from one phase to the other is accompanied by the need to find new skills and abilities in accordance with the fresh life circumstances that a life cycle transition imposes. The life cycle does not stop with the end of adolescence for there are adult life cycle transitions which may or may not be associated with extrinsic life events such as bereavement, change of marital partner and events in the families of origin of the parents. The more family members as individuals are going through critical transitions the more the family will be stressed. In family therapy theory, symptoms are defined as both the expression of the stress that life cycle transitions impose on the family, and the demands for adaptation and change that are required by it (Haley 1973). They are seen as manifestations of attempts, serving the whole family's needs, to slow down or to alleviate the consequences of life cycle transitions.

(iv) The assessment of the interactional structure of the family is the most characteristic activity of the family therapist as diagnostician. It can only be carried out by a careful survey of the non-verbal and verbal interaction of the family when seen together. This includes the pattern of communication; the structure and strengths of coalitions and alliances; of how intergenerational boundaries are defined and set up; the modes of nurturance and control, and the way individuality and cohesiveness are given place in the family. The therapist makes these assessments during the discussion of the presenting problems. As the therapist observes patterns he can adjust the nature of the negotiation around the definition of the problem in order to test out elements as he sees them.

The accumulation of all these different strands in the understanding of the family can be put together as a family hypothesis. This is an answer, in part, to the question: why does this family at this phase of its life cycle, given its socio-ethnic origins and its family history as we know it, seem to need to function with this symptom? What 'problems' of the whole family are solved by the presenting problem? What are the risks for the individual members of the family if the presenting 'patient' did not have the 'problems'? It will be seen that such an hypothesis is very different from the formulation of other mental health practices within which the problem is seen in terms of the individual as a psychobiological entity sensitive to social pressures. The family therapy formulation carries with it a view of the family as having a pattern which family functioning seeks to perpetuate. It is a general principle of family therapy that the family will resist attempts to change the pattern of family life and that symptoms are an expression both of the distress that a particular pattern of family life may engender but are also processes which enhance continuity in family patterns.

4 Interventions in family therapy

Interventions in family therapy are devised to change the pattern of family life. The family members are distressed and, to a lesser or greater extent, affected by the symptoms, and this is the motivation for change. This is facilitated if the family members feel that the family therapist has a genuine wish to enhance the wellbeing of each of them, and has respect for the investment each has in the family.

In general, simpler problems are treated as though they were manifestations of a failure of control in the family, *as if* they were unwitting misbehaviour. These treatments often look like fairly simple behavioural control techniques but in fact they are directed at changing the pattern of family interaction, usually by enhancing the effectiveness of parental control and increasing the differentiation of parent and child functions. It is usual for these behavioural techniques to include an attempt to develop the strength of the parents, if there are two parents, as a system ('parental sub-system') and to increase the sense of cohesiveness in the offspring group ('child sub-system'). As symptoms come under control, or their resistiveness to coming under control are manifest, and as the family's commitment to the therapy increases, the therapy becomes more openly directed towards changing those aspects of the pattern of family life which seem to be maintained by and are maintaining the presenting symptom. Gentle confrontation, role playing, sculpting and task setting may all be used in this phase of the treatment to help the family devise new methods of relating to each other in ways appropriate to the phase of development of the family life cycle, entry to which is prevented by the symptom.

It is unusual for straightforward 'interpretation' to be effective and appropriate, although aspects of paradoxical injunctions, advising against changing the symptoms at all, or at least not in anything like the immediate future, may function as interpretations. In family therapy an expression by the therapist of his or her understanding of the family problem early on in the treatment is likely to increase the family's resistance and is therefore contra-indicated.

At all stages of the therapy the therapist must maintain, on balance, a neutral relationship with the family; although from time to time the therapist may seem to be taking sides with one or other family member or one or other sub-system this should only be for strategic purposes. It should soon be followed by an apparent side-taking in the opposite direction. As a rule, the principle of 'positive connotation', whereby the therapist attempts to understand what is going on as well-meant and benign, should be sustained. The family should never feel that there is any continuing blame from the therapist to any one member of the family for the problems within the family.

Special Features in the Family Therapy of Adolescence

In the engagement process with families containing an adolescent the therapist must usually be especially careful not to be seen to be taking sides with either the adolescent or the parents. Adolescent problems frequently produce some sort of reminiscences within therapists of their own adolescent experiences, which leads them to feel either over-identified with the young person striving for independence, or to be excessively aligned with the parents experiencing the disruption and apparent destabilisation of the family that adolescence often seems to perpetrate. The therapist should express empathic understanding of the apparent 'plight' of the adolescent being pushed forward as the patient; but at no time should this go against an equally forceful and effective demonstration of the therapist's awareness of the parents' wish to maintain control of their lives and household, and their bewilderment and puzzlement as to what their youngster is going through. It is especially important that the therapist recognises how frightened and out of control an adolescent feels when his or her parents feel, somehow, disqualified by the adolescent's condition from exercising appropriate parental authority. At the same time it is important to recognise that the adolescent is alarmed by the apparent threat to his autonomy that an augmentation of parental control would produce.

An adolescent family member, who is in the position of the symptom bearer, will frequently be un-cooperative to the point of mutiny. He may refuse to enter the interview room, or will sit with his back to the rest of the family. The therapist will often have to announce that it is clear that the adolescent feels that it would be wrong to contribute to the discussions of the problem and that, therefore, for the time being there should be no pressure to do so. It is crucial, as early as possible, for the therapist to attempt to redefine the presenting symptoms in terms of the disturbance of the normal process of increasing independence and separate identity development which goes on in adolescence, but without making it seem to be any sort of criticism of the family.

Again, there are cultural effects to be aware of. Spiegel (1967; 1968) pointed out that there are different rates of adoption of the 'host culture' in different family members of migrant people. A mother who may not learn the language of the country to which the family migrates, and who mixes with her own ethnic group, may know very little about the expectations, within the host culture, for adolescent development. Her husband, out at work, may mix more with the host culture and may develop some understanding of expectations about adolescence in the country to which they have migrated, and may even have the idea of taking on some of those expectations. Children going to school in the host culture are highly affected by the peer culture. Adherence by adolescents to their peer culture leads them to have wishes for levels of independence and freedom which are common within their peer group, and this can cause disputes with parents. It may be no coincidence that mixtures of perhaps relatively unusual cultural origins seem to be found within the parents of youngsters who are admitted to the adolescent unit. Different and even contradictory expectations about the nature of the adolescent *passage* between the two parents and different members of the sibship may need to be understood in terms of these sociocultural differences, and are part of the family diagnosis of an adolescent disorder. As is often attested, the process of adolescent development in the younger generation of the family stimulates the parents or parent to re-experience their own adolescent strivings and, perhaps, conflicts. The relationship which pertained between the parents and their own parents, the grandparents, at the time that the parents were going through adolescent development may be seen in part to shape parental attitudes to their own adolescence. Premature precipitation into excessive autonomy as an outcome of illness, death or disappearance in the grandparental generation may lead parents to feel that there is an end to the possibility of their being able to be useful parents to their growing up children. Parents are, commonly, under the influence of a conscious determination not to impose on their own offspring the worse aspects of their own adolescence. This can leave them with a certainty as to how they are not to behave, but an uncertainty as to how they can behave. Continuing strife between a single parent and one or other grandparent may also be a clear impingement on the life of the adolescent who is presented as a patient.

There is a 'complication' of the life cycle when a parent attempting a major shift in the direction of his own life does so at a time which coincides with serious uncertainties in self-assessment within the adolescent. The unconscious or sometimes conscious apprehension on the part of the whole family as to how the parents can manage without children to look after is a regular feature, too, of families containing an adolescent psychiatric patient. The symptom is then understandable, in family therapy terms, as a way of protecting the parents from experiencing the post-parenting phase (the 'empty-nest' syndrome of Dare, 1982a). Apparently regressive adolescent symptoms can be seen as functioning to halt movement in a family within which parenting is seen as the main function of the first generation of the family, and when there is an accompanying belief that the marital aspect of the spouse relationship will not be sufficiently strong to sustain the family as an entity. Adolescent siblings, like all the other family members, may suffer from the belief that the parents need a little child for their relationship to be harmonious and for the family to have an existence. Regressive symptoms in an adolescent, such as severe school phobia, anorexia nervosa, severe obsessional neurosis and even functional psychoses may have the *effect* of keeping the parental task as one of caring for an apparently younger child. Here, it is important to note, there need be no aetiological connotation of such a treatment. Because the symptom seems to serve a function as part of the family's problem of accepting a life cycle transition, it does not in any way infer that the symptom is caused by that need. This is an especially important consideration in the psychoses, where any sense of the family therapist elucidating causation can easily seem like blaming the parents for an extremely serious condition. Although family therapists may harbour convictions that there is a causative relationship between family functioning and pathology in the adolescent, it is usually a serious technical error to express such a belief to the family. Despite any views to the contrary that the family therapist has, it is quite inappropriate to imply that the family's *hypothesised need* for the symptom is a *cause* for the symptom. In fact it can be important for the therapist to make an explicit announcement to the family that there is no certain knowledge about the origins of the symptom and that the therapist does not believe the family to be responsible for causing the symptom. The therapist must emphasise the belief that the family may be able to find resources to help the youngster in distress. The purpose of the therapy is to enhance this possibility rather than to seek for causes. Such a statement is strategically useful for the development of an appropriate working relationship, and for diminishing the handicapping levels of guilt that belief in their own responsibility for causing the disorder may engender. It is also professionally honest.

The interactional characteristics of families containing an adolescent who presents as a patient are diverse. Features that are apparently characteristic of families containing an anorexic youngster have been described by Minuchin (1975, 1978) whilst Harbin has tried to identify features common to families containing a violent adolescent (Harbin, 1983). Hirsch & Leff (1975) attempted to replicate the findings by Wynne and his co-workers (1958) of particular communication patterns in families containing a young schizophrenic patient, without success. However, in subsequent work Leff (1979) has been able to show that there are features in the communication of affect within families containing a schizophrenic patient which in some instances are associated with relapse, and which are capable of being changed by treatment regimes including appropriate family interventions. Future research, it is hoped, should increase the specificity of family therapists' understandings of family interactions in different disorders. There is, however, no particular reason why psychiatric syndromes identified on the basis of the phenomenology of individual patients should have clearly differentiable family disturbances. For example, in a study of the expressed emotion within families containing an anorexic patient there are features which are not dissimilar to those found within families containing a schizophrenic patient. Although Leff (1979) has shown that high levels of expressed emotion predict relapse in schizophrenic patients who return home there is no evidence, as yet, that this is so for anorectic youngsters; however, we have some evidence that some levels of expressed emotion in families containing an anorectic youngster predict drop-out from family therapy. (Szmukler et al 1985).

Methods of intervention with families containing an adolescent patient do not differ in any systematic way from the general techniques of family therapy. Such symptoms among younger adolescents as self-starvation, school refusal, obsessional behaviours and stealing within the family are, in general, potentially amenable to an initial strategy of parental control of symptoms. The older the adolescent, the less appropriate control techniques become, and the more strategic, paradoxical working out of the family's problems is required. Adolescent inpatients have often been placed beyond the reach of parental symptom management, and alternative forms of family therapy are needed.

Problems of Family Therapy with Families Containing an Adolescent Youngster in an Inpatient Unit

All the foregoing has addressed the general issue of family therapy with families containing an adolescent. This is necessary as it is so much the subject-matter of the consultations between a family therapist and an inpatient unit. It has also been necessary to outline the general principles of family therapy with adolescence in order to clarify why there must be considerable problems in mobilising family therapy for inpatients. Nonetheless Ro-Trock (Ro-Trock et al, 1977) was able to show that family therapy as an adjunct to the inpatient milieu was capable of improving the efficacy of the overall programme. Clinical experience at the adolescent unit has shown that family therapy can also, under some circumstances, replace inpatient admission for certain relatively serious conditions, eg. anorexia nervosa, (Dare 1982b).

Overall, it has seemed that family therapy is a very useful part of the inpatient regime, and staff have continued to use it with a significant proportion of the families of inpatients in the Adolescent Unit at the Bethlem Royal Hospital.

Haley in his monograph on adolescent problems (1980) suggested that in order to function effectively with a family containing a youngster who was an inpatient, the family therapist had to have control over the admission or discharge of the youngster. The experiences reported here do not sustain this. Throughout the time of the family therapy consultations the family therapy consultant has had no administrative or executive authority within the adolescent unit; this has remained with the staff of the unit. Bruggen (1973; 1982) has been running a unit for many years on principles which wholeheartedly take a family therapy approach. This does not, in any way, pertain in the Adolescent Unit at the Bethlem Royal Hospital. The problems for mobilising family therapy in an inpatient unit which is not run by a family therapist on family therapy principles must be clarified, in order to identify the role of the family therapy consultant in facilitating the possibility of inpatient adolescents benefiting in the way that Ro-Trock has shown.

Psychiatric practice seeks to define the nature and prognosis of disorders in patients under the care of the psychiatrist. Organic, developmental, psychopathological, family factors and wider social factors may all be hypothesised as causative multi-factorial aetiological features. These aetiological frameworks will carry with them specific implications for pharmacological, psychological, educational, milieu and other remedies. The theory of family therapy in no way seeks to deny the importance of these aetiological propositions, but addresses itself to other issues. All disorders are assumed to be capable of being influenced by changes in family life. Although the theory of family therapy does not need to imply a family cause for, for example, schizophrenia, it would predict that a youngster with schizophrenia would be in great difficulties in moving through adolescence. These difficulties may be maintained by family processes which need not, necessarily, be substantially different from the family processes which seem to be relevant to the inhibition of adolescent development in, for example, severe school phobia.

The family therapist would not expect to have a part to play in the specific pharmacological or individual psychotherapeutic issues addressed in the care of the individual patient. These are the business of others. The problem, for the family therapist, is that the mobilisation of the other forms of therapy with their aetiological implications communicate information to the family and wider social network as to the nature of the suffering of the youngster. That communication endorses the generally held view that psychological problems are uniquely the property of the individual suffering from the problems. They imply that responsibility for the process of change resides either within the patient, or in the hands of the professionals. A family can quite reasonably believe that they cannot be responsible for effecting biochemical changes in the brain of their offspring. Nor need they feel any responsibility for such putative biochemical disturbances. Similarly, although differently, an individual psychotherapist or a behaviour therapist must identify processes within the individual patient which can, with the patient's cooperation, be affected by the therapist's intervention. An individual psychotherapist, especially, must maximise the extent to which the individual patient himself feels responsible for his own situation so that he can find ways to change it. The family therapist wants to help the family discover abilities to change their own relationship pattern so that the disruption of family life and the failure to move appropriately through adolescent development can be overcome.

The whole process of identifying the nature of the disorder in the individual patient, and of inculcating them into the ward regime, may suggest strongly to the family that they may no longer be in any way responsible for their youngster. There is a very natural and understandable tendency for families to believe that an inpatient unit will function to 'cure' their youngster so that he is returned to the bosom of the family more like the family would want him to be. General family work may have to alter erroneous expectations about the extent of therapeutic change in the course of a ward admission but the family therapist's activity with the family will be radically different. The family therapist cannot, usually, go along with the family's belief that the ward staff are 'curing' the patient. The family have to be helped to alter some of their perceptions of the nature of the problem in order that they may be motivated to change their own pattern of life. This is very rarely welcomed, even under the best of circumstances. When the family find that they themselves are being asked to change, they immediately feel that far from being relieved of the burden and worry of their disturbed youngster they are being asked to take responsibility for him. Under these circumstances the family therapist has to use a great deal of forceful mobilisation of sympathy, care and resourceful re-framing of problems in order to develop any form of therapeutic alliance with the family.

The Role of the Family Therapy Consultant

A large part of the job of the family therapy consultant is to hear the story of the inpatient and the family, in order to make assessments and supervise the development of sensible interventions out of acceptable hypotheses. Much of this task has the form of any family therapy supervision and can use any of the following formats: verbal case presentations, live observation, video recording of sessions, role play or sculpting of families by the consultation group, and consultation with outside workers involved in the unit's families. The hypotheses developed must be conceptually congruent with the established habits of thought of the consultation group, and the therapeutic interventions suggested must be adapted to the qualities and characteristics of the therapists.

The consultant must constantly be creative in carrying forward the thinking of the ward staff. As the longstanding members of the consultation group develop in their own professional skills, they inevitably incorporate aspects of the consultant's thinking into their contributions to case discussions away from the family therapy consultation. This may be welcomed in the unit generally, but it is inevitable that it will also produce some dissonance with the culture of the ward. The consultant must be very careful not to be thought of as setting up an alternative ideology, challenging the established culture. The consultant must put forward those different points of view which make the family therapy a real enhancement of the ward's therapeutic work, but he must make sure that there is never any disrespect for the points of view, working styles and contributions outside of the family therapy consultation group. The consultant should always ask about the overall diagnostic view of the ward team, about the reasons for admission, and about the overall span and plan of treatment.

It inevitably happens that even in asking such straightforward questions the family therapy consultant may identify tensions around differences of opinions. The consultant can notice these, openly, being sure not to take sides in major differences, and should 'place' his own observations so as to minimise the incorporation of the family therapy viewpoint into conflicting bodies of opinions. This may sound to be idealising the function of the consultant, but in fact it is only an example of habitual family therapy technique whereby interventions are *'placed'* admist the family in such a way as to accept and clarify the existing and necessary managerial hierarchy. The consultant is no more seeking to make junior staff subservient *or* rebellious, any more than he is seeking these attitudes in the offspring sub-system *vis à vis* the parental sub-system in the practice of family therapy. The family therapist should insert his point of view, recommending it, but making it clear that the consultation group need to feel it is congruent and helpful for themselves, just as opinions or tasks are offered to families in therapy.

The consultant should, in this way, be able to demonstrate some of the skills of the therapy by the way the consultation is conducted. He should accept that his job is only to point out the family structure, as he understands it, and to suggest ways of using such understanding therapeutically, if it fits with the overall plan. There is no reason why the therapist should not point out how points of view and requirements from other inputs into the unit are discrepant with the family therapy point of view. The limitations or restrictions that other aspects of management place on the possibilities of family therapy being effective may need to be identified and expressed. The deleterious effects that the proposed family therapy interventions, if instituted, could have on the rest of the management plan can also be discussed. The consultation group should always be urged to refer the conclusions of the family therapy discussions to management meetings.

Frequently, staff members conducting the family therapy can take part in management meetings, receiving information and even instructions from other staff, without causing problems for their therapeutic role with the family. Occasionally, other staff members, feeling strongly about the interactions between the family, the patient and the ward, want to have a point of view expressed in the family about the patient's prognosis or medical management, or want the family confronted with their apparently harmful effects on the patient. Being the spokesman for views from management meetings is at times destructive of the family therapy. On hearing something of this, the consultant should encourage the group to think through how an appropriate division of roles could be negotiated.

Summary

Over many years, a family therapy consultation has been conducted with a multi-disciplinary staff group. The aim has been to facilitate mobilisation of a family therapy framework and the implementation of the practice of family therapy as part of the adolescent unit's eclectic approach. The chapter describes the theoretical frameworks and practical techniques used within the consultation. The assessment of the impact of the consultation on the unit's functioning is beyond the scope of the chapter.

References and Further Reading

Bruggen P, Byng-Hall J & Pitt-Aikens T (1973) The reason for admission as a focus of work for an adolescent unit. *British Journal of Psychiatry*, 122, 319-329

Bruggen P & O'Brian C (1982) An adolescent unit's focus on family admission decisions. In H T Harbin (ed) *The Psychiatric Hospital and the Family*. NY: Spectrum Publications

Dare C (1982a) The empty nest: families with older adolescents and the models of family therapy. Ch 18, 353-360. In A Bentovim, G Gorrell-Barnes & A Cooklin (eds) *Family Therapy*, 2. London: Academic Press

Dare C (1982b) Family therapy for families containing an anorectic youngster. Paper presented at the 4th Ross Conference on Medical Research, November 1982.

Erikson E H (1959) *Identity and the Life Cycle*. New York: International Universities Press

Gorrell-Barnes G (1984) Systems theory and family theory. Ch 13, 216-229. In L Hersov & M Rutter (eds) *Child Psychiatry: Modern Approaches*. Oxford: Blackwell Publications

Haley J (1973) *Uncommon Therapy*. New York: W W Norton

Haley J (1980) *Leaving Home*. New York: McGraw Hill

Harbin H T & Madden D J (1983) Assaultive adolescents: family decision-making parameters. *Family Process*, 22, 109-118

Hirsch S R, Leff J P (1975) *Abnormalities in Parents of Schizophrenics*. Maudsley Monograph No. 22. Oxford University Press

Leff J P (1979) Developments in family treatment of schizophrenia. *Psychiatric Quarterly*, 51, 216-232

Minuchin S, Baker L, Rosman B, Liebman R, Milman L & Todd T (1975) A conceptual model of psychosomatic illness in children. *Archives of General Psychiatry*, 32, 1031-1038

Minuchin S, Rosman B & Baker L (1978) *Psychosomatic Families*. Cambridge: Harvard University Press

Ro-Trock C, Wellisch D & Schroder J (1977) A family therapy outcome study in an in-patient setting. *American Journal of Orthopsychiatry*, 47, 514-522

Spiegel J P (1957, rev 1968) The resolution of role conflict within the family. Ch 30, 391-411. In N W Bell, E F Vogel (eds) *A Modern Introduction to the Family*. New York: The Free Press.

Szmukler G, Eisler I, Russell G, Dare C (1985) Anorexia nervosa, parental 'expressed emotion' and dropping out of treatment. British Journal of Psychiatry, 147, 265-271

Spiegel J P (1968) Cultural strain, family role patterns, and intrapsychic conflict. Ch 15. 367–389. In J G Howell (ed) *Theory and Practice of Family Psychiatry*. Edinburgh: Oliver Boyd

Wynne L C, Ryckoff I M, Day J & Hirsch S I (1958) Pseudo-mutuality in the family relations of schizophrenics. *Psychiatry*, **21**, 205–220

Yule W, Steinberg D, Ryle R & Dare C (1983) Techniques of consultation. *Newsletter of the Association of Child Psychology, Psychiatry and Allied Disciplines*

The Adolescent Unit
Edited by Derek Steinberg
© 1986 D. Steinberg

10 Individual Psychotherapy in a Residential Setting

Peter Wilson

Equipped with a degree in industrial economics, I began working life as an unattached youth worker. After three years I trained in social work at the London School of Economics where I was impressed by the psychoanalytic viewpoint and by Winnicott's and Stuart Prince's teaching there. I then worked as a psychiatric caseworker at Hawthorne Cedar Knolls School, a residential treatment centre for children in New York. This was a stimulating, challenging and invigorating period for me; the atmosphere and the in-service training were influential on my ideas about the applications of psychoanalysis. While I was in New York I heard about the Hampstead Child Therapy Clinic, directed by Anna Freud, and returned to England to train there for four years, an experience which included a personal analysis and supervised analytic work with children, as well as the time and opportunity to study psychoanalytic theory. Since qualifying there in 1971 I have spent most of my time trying to apply what I learned to the problems of working psychotherapeutically with children, adolescents and their families in child guidance clinics, a walk-in centre for adolescents (the Brent Consultation Centre) and at the Maudsley and Bethlem Royal Hospitals, where I have been increasingly involved with teaching, supervision and consultative work. My experience as consultant at Peper Harow Therapeutic Community and at the Adolescent Inpatient Unit at Bethlem has focussed my interest on the place of individual psychotherapy within a variety of clinical approaches and contexts.

———◆———

DS Peter, you come here regularly on a Wednesday morning and meet a dozen or so of us. There are people from all the different disciplines, mostly with very different experience and backgrounds, and all with quite different types of involvement with the patients we'll be discussing. There will be the adolescents' psychotherapists, and their supervisors. There will also be their teachers; their doctors; there will be some living with them practically *in loco parentis*, some working with their actual parents and families. That's quite a crowd, and we all want to learn something about a piece of psychotherapy, and something about psychotherapy in general. It strikes me as being very different from the ordinary notion of 'psychotherapy supervision'.

97

PW Well, I suppose 'ordinary' psychotherapy supervision takes place most comfortably in outpatient settings. Clinicians bring material from sessions with adolescents who attend more or less regularly and who are well enough to get along in the community. Under these conditions supervision can proceed in a fairly orderly and circumscribed way. External circumstances may be important; they may be thought about and talked about but the focus is on what the adolescent brings into the sessions; on what he chooses to talk about, and how he relates to the therapist. The supervisor and therapist are thinking about the internal life of the adolescent; how he sees life and how he feels about it and how he feels about himself; what it all means to him as he carries it about from one place to another and into the psychotherapy sessions. They work on the assumption that what exists and occurs in the psychotherapy session reflects what is going on elsewhere; the sessions are taken as a kind of microcosm of the adolescent's life in general.

Now the seed of that idea prevails in individual psychotherapy everywhere, and in this unit, too; with some adolescents here, it does occur, particularly in the later stages of their time here. But in general, the situation here is quite different. This is a complex setting. The adolescents are severely disturbed. Attempts to help them function outside have failed. When they arrive, they are usually in a terrible state. Some have attempted suicide, or have mutilated or starved themselves; some ruminate and ritualise obsessionally, to the point of practically coming to a standstill. Some act impulsively, recklessly or violently. They are not, to put it mildly, easy to treat. And they don't settle agreeably to formal individual psychotherapy. The clinicians and the teachers here are faced with confusion; with powerful, upsetting, puzzling emotions, fantasies, behaviour. They have to think and cope as best they can, use a whole variety of strategies, and individual psychotherapy has to take its place in the midst of all this. It's not the exclusive treatment. It has to be considered in context, with reference to what is going on around. So too does psychotherapy supervision.

DS Suppose for a moment we stay with the 'ordinary' model of psychotherapy and psychotherapy supervision. How important is it to know what the adolescent is doing outside the sessions; or about the effect he is having on other people? He may well choose not to let you know about all that in the sessions. Don't the staff bring along two sorts of information? They bring along stories about what the youngster has been up to. But they also bring along their feelings. It seems to me the sort of information an adolescent's family, teachers, even friends, would bring to an individual psychotherapy supervision session if they could.

PW I think that's right. The nurses in a sense act as parents. They are very close to what is going on. So, too, are the teachers, more so than the teachers in an ordinary secondary school. What you're asking is how this information influences the individual psychotherapy; or would the psychotherapist be better off not knowing? That's an important issue. It applies to the psychotherapist, to the supervisor and to myself as consultant.

DS Then are you helped or hindered by all this extra material?

PW In a way, both. It's a split answer. In pure terms, all that kind of information can be an intrusion, a nuisance. It can have the effect of cluttering up the psychotherapist's thinking, taking his mind off the essential job of tuning into the adolescent's inner state. You can start picking up the anxiety of parents, teachers, nurses; their irritation, exasperation, their anger. Sometimes, too, you can be swayed by their idealisation, an over-eagerness to come to the defence of the adolescent. You might well find yourself identifying with them; or against them. You aren't unfettered and open to what the adolescent is trying to say to you or how he wants to make use of you. You become lumbered with other people's anxieties, expectations, even enthusiasms. Your perception of the adolescent can be clouded; so too can be your own responses.

DS That would apply to the psychotherapeutic work itself, as well as to the supervision and consultation sessions?

PW Yes. It would. All this other information can be an interference at any level of the work. A bit of me would not want to know about all the rest. So that I, as therapist, as supervisor or as consultant, have my space, my setting, my boundary – the conditions of work where I would like just to focus on the adolescent and try and listen very attentively and exclusively to what matters to him, and to no one else. These are conditions, too, I might say, that the adolescent might want for himself; to have someone impartial, outside the hurly-burly of immediate life, not associated too closely with all the others who impinge on him.

In putting it this way I'm acknowledging a certain extreme line; a purist position in order to clarify a point. Ultimately, such a position would be for my own convenience and advantage; to give room in my mind to be receptive to what is inside the adolescent, to have the space to form my *own* impressions in response to the adolescent. It's about preserving a special, separate, distinct individual psychotherapy setting; important for the therapist and I think for the individual adolescent.

DS But from what you've been saying this position is not realistic; it isn't possible in an inpatient unit. Individual psychotherapy can't exist here in isolation: the clinicians who do psychotherapy here are part of the unit; they are about the place; they know and discuss things with other staff; the adolescents see them around outside the sessions. And many of our adolescents don't respond positively to the offer of formal regular individual treatment sessions. That's why some of them are in the unit in the first place.

PW All true. Nothing is cut and dried, least of all with disturbed adolescents; the position I was describing is perfectionist. It's a useful yardstick, but it has to be adapted. It seems to me that working with children and adolescents, working with a wide range of disorders and working in residential establishments requires a preparedness to compromise with an ideal psychotherapeutic model. This was a model that was originally created out of the constructions and developments of psychoanalysis. In that model, certain procedures and conditions were established to facilitate free association and the uncovering and interpretation of unconscious conflicts. The treatment was also of course undertaken initially with adults; they were motivated, seeking to relieve their own distress; they were articulate and ready and able to co-operate. It was conducted in private, separate from everyday life.

That was the model; and it is and should be practised with certain adults and with some children and adolescents. It is, in my view, a very profound and effective treatment with certain people. It is not applicable, nor even appropriate, to everyone and not, as far as I can see, to many of the adolescents whom we try to help in this unit. Yet, the persuasiveness of the model persists; and I find that many clinical workers, particularly those newly interested in individual psychotherapy, believe that this is the real thing, *the* way of doing psychotherapy, however impracticable it is or how resistant the adolescent may be.

So I come back to the other side of the split answer. It can be an encumbrance to have to contend with other people's information and feelings; and yet it is necessary. There is a constant tension in psychotherapy with young disturbed adolescents; you have to hold on to some degree of analytic distance, and yet acknowledge and adapt to the crises, rapid changes, risks and dangers that occur in their actual lives with their families and those working with them. As you say, that's part of the reality about why they're in hospital. It seems to me there is no absolute solution to that kind of tension; what occurs is a kind of compromised process. You really cannot divorce yourself from what is going on around your psychotherapy sessions. If concerned people are anxious and feel helpless about an adolescent attempting suicide or putting himself into dangerous situations; or if they find themselves having to cope with agitated and extreme behaviour, they have a right to communicate that to the psycho-therapist. They might think, rightly or wrongly, that this has been aroused by the psychotherapy. The psychotherapist cannot disclaim responsibility. To put it another way, I don't think you can conduct psychotherapy with a young adolescent, whether on an outpatient or inpatient basis, unless you have got the support and co-operation of those around him. Their sanction is essential; and if they feel cut off from you, because you don't listen to their concerns, that may well undermine the psychotherapy, one way or another.

DS   That makes sense. Is that the main reason for talking and listening to teachers, nurses, parents – to keep them comfortable, as it were, to ensure support for individual psychotherapy? Or does the psychotherapist benefit from listening to these other people? Given everything you've said about hindrances, is the psychotherapist also helped by knowing what other people say and feel about the adolescent?

PW Yes. In most cases, the psychotherapy can be facilitated, moved along more quickly. Again, I come back to the question of adapting the original psychoanalytic model; adapting it to special circumstances such as inpatient units; and to people at a particular developmental phase – early adolescence – and those with particularly severe emotional and conduct disorders. With young adolescents you cannot expect, to say the least, free association. Often you cannot even expect acknowledgement of internal distress or a clear wish to explore feelings and thoughts. Even where that wish may exist, with some self-awareness, there may not be the readiness or the capacity to put things into words; nor much comprehension of the idea or purpose of psychotherapy. When an adolescent says 'I don't know' about what he feels – a phrase we hear only too often and wearily – he means it. The material may be sparse, too. There may be silence. Sessions may be missed or interrupted; the adolescent may walk out, and so on. Even where the adolescent is engaged, talking, trying to work something out, he may well be selective; sometimes simply forgetting painful experiences that have happened in the unit, or wanting to avoid thinking about them, because he feels bad, ashamed or confused, dreads ridicule or rejection. The adolescent may want to keep the psychotherapist ignorant; or keep him benign, to at least not spoil one relationship in the unit.

Where this sort of thing is going on, individual psychotherapy may well proceed slowly and at a tangent to what is important. Significant, disturbing happenings may be occurring in the adolescent's life that are not being mentioned, let alone explored. If the psychotherapist is not aware of them from other sources, the psychotherapy may go along in a vacuum, sealed off, unreal. The adolescent may feel he's getting away with something; he may feel frightened that he can deceive or trick the psychotherapist. He may lose respect in the psychotherapist or feel worthless himself. More fundamentally, he may feel unsafe and uncared for, that the psychotherapist seems so indifferent or ill-informed. As far as the adolescent is concerned, in an inpatient unit the psychotherapist is a member of the staff; he assumes that the psychotherapist knows what is going on.

DS Can you give some examples of what you need to know?

PW It's important, for example, that the psychotherapist knows if the adolescent has tried to kill or hurt himself; whether he's run away or been involved in a bad fight; whether he has returned from time at home in a disturbed state; whether his mood has been depressed, or animated; whether he's formed a particular relationship; who else has he being talking to. Those sort of things, I would think, in most cases, are necessary information for an individual psychotherapist in an inpatient unit. Without it he may be ludicrously in the dark; unhelpful to himself, and to the adolescent. I'm thinking of a recent instance where a boy who, the night before his session, had hidden a daypatient, a girl, in his room. He had strongly identified with the girl's despair, her ambivalence towards her mother and her wish to run away; he had wanted to protect the girl. When he was found out he felt furious and useless. Just before the session, the nurse had wanted to inform the psychotherapist about all this. The therapist, holding to the notion of preserving some therapeutic distance, thought it best not to listen to such information at that time. The result was a long, difficult, silent session, in which the possibility for some exploration of the adolescent's feelings about the whole incident, immediate from the night before, was almost lost. The adolescent felt confused and, I would think, unsafe with a psychotherapist, a member of staff, who appeared not to know what had happened. I also wondered about the effect of the psychotherapist's apparent indifference to the nurse's information; how far the nurse was left feeling devalued, unheard and potentially resistant to co-operating with the individual psychotherapy.

How the psychotherapist uses this kind of information in individual sessions is another matter. It's impossible here to prescribe *the* way. Every case is different. In terms of general approach, a fundamental principle should be followed. And that is simply to set out in every session to wait, follow, observe and listen; to open the session up, by giving space and time to the adolescent to fill as he must; to pay respect to where the adolescent is and to see what he brings. The psychotherapist's attentiveness in that moment is sacred. But it may well be, in view of the adolescent's difficulty in conveying what is important, that the psychotherapist's 'outside' knowledge will give him that extra clue, that extra idea, that will enable him to clamber through the confusion and say or think something relevant. The psychotherapist will be able to introduce what he knows from elsewhere in the context of what the adolescent is saying, or how he is being with the psychotherapist in that session. He will also be able to understand the silence.

DS You tell the patient what you've heard?

PW I'm not particularly in favour of an instant confrontation – you know, the psychotherapist kicking off with a list of wrongs and ills and the demand to know what it's all about. But when you're left with a blank, a flat denial, even when you've looked and waited for sensitive openings, I think it is appropriate to bring in information that's important; to register reality, to underline the seriousness of whatever is going on, to convey concern and interest. It's honest. If psychotherapy is to have any validity, it must be an attempt at honesty, the truth. The adolescent must sense that the therapist is straight.

DS What about information in the other direction? From the psychotherapist to the other people involved with the adolescent? It makes me wonder about confidentiality, and about privacy.

PW In an inpatient unit, and even more generally outside in work with children and young adolescents, complete confidentiality is a myth. It cannot be absolute; it's not possible. Children and adolescents are dependent on adults who take care of them and need to know the dangers. Children and adolescents themselves don't believe any such promise of total confidentiality. There is an assumption, even I would say a wish, that parents, staff, 'know'. They care enough to talk to each other. They may seem to want to keep things secret, or secure a confidante, but they also take a certain kind of comfort in the knowledge or the fantasy that parents or caretakers bother enough to think about them and share knowledge about them. Of course, they grumble and protest about staff gossiping and ganging up, 'you can't trust anyone around here', that sort of thing. But ultimately, I believe, they feel contained.

So it's not an issue that alarms me, that rigidifies me. There are things the psychotherapist has to communicate to other staff. I'm thinking, for example, of the very depressed girl, preoccupied with killing herself, with worthlessness, with self hatred, becoming particularly despairing in a session. It was essential that the psychotherapist notified the nursing staff of the girl's state of mind and intentions, to ensure that they kept a close eye on her. There are so many other examples of destructive or self-destructive possibilities, of running away, of taking drugs, and when you are into an area your colleagues need to know about, of course you make it clear to the adolescent that you must inform others. Of course, there is then the risk that the adolescent will withhold things. But on balance, in an inpatient unit, that is the lesser risk.

So we have a two-way sharing of experience, in the child's interests. But at its best it also does much to demystify individual psychotherapy, to reduce fantasy that can be the source of envy and can be quite off-beam. It is also an important way of teaching about feelings. When, for example, the psychotherapist can give some idea of how he is experiencing the adolescent, of feeling denigrated, frightened, useless, as a reflection of what the adolescent is feeling inside; then this becomes something that belongs to the whole unit; it is live material, potentially useful to everyone, not something remote, hidden, irrelevant.

DS Which material would be kept private? How do you decide?

PW It's a difficult issue. Like so much else it's a question of balance and judgement. Putting it in broad terms it has to do with what is communal, to be shared; and what is individual, to be kept private. The psychotherapist is part of the team, however much he might want to set himself apart. Yet he is accountable also to the adolescent, to treat him as an individual in his own right. The adolescent is his own person; yet he too is part of a group. What he does affects others, and vice versa. A disorganised, fragmented, disruptive adolescent creates widespread concern; there is a communal need to mobilise all resources and this includes information. The psychotherapist plays his part in this. Other adolescents are more self-contained, and their questions and fears more open to help in a contained way, contained within the psychotherapy session; I'm thinking about sexual ideas, wishes, fantasies, ambivalence about parents, alive or lost, preoccupations about the body, doubts and despair about the self, about ever becoming a happy or successful adult. And all the feelings, attitudes and expectations that arise in relation to the therapist. These are largely private matters. They are not, in my view, the business of everybody. They need some space for reflection and experimentation. Adolescents hate to be exposed and tied down to passing thoughts, resolutions, declarations. They need someone to understand this transience. This too doesn't need to be shared; nor am I convinced that other staff would want to have it.

A final point; it goes without saying that everybody in an adolescent unit should treat information, shared or private, with respect; to guard against needless gossip or abusing what one knows in moments of anger and retaliation.

DS I'm sometimes taken by surprise by what a relatively inexperienced member of staff brings to one of the consultation sessions; perhaps a junior nurse or a teacher, someone without much in the way of experience in psychotherapy. Suddenly there's the realisation that something very important is going on between that member of staff and the adolescent, and meanwhile the proper psychotherapist is stuck. This raises two questions for me. Firstly, the status of work that is based on a relationship between a member of staff and a patient, and which is getting somewhere with exploring and helping the adolescent's problems; but which isn't based on psychotherapeutic training. Is that psychotherapy? The second question is about the problem of the adolescent spreading his problems all over the place instead of bringing them to a regular session with the same person. Isn't it important to encourage that boy to take things back to the designated person, even though he says he can talk more easily to this or that person?

PW I've been mildly amused by that sort of thing in the Wednesday sessions. We have the registrar puffing away, struggling to be a psychotherapist with a refractory adolescent, and then hearing, almost by chance, that the adolescent has formed a close attachment with, say, a nurse or a teacher and is talking about everything that mattered in his life.

Of course, it's a problem for the designated psychotherapist, and that needs attention and respect. But it's also unfortunate if the other member of staff didn't think or didn't know that what he or she is doing is important; that it is not part of his assigned job, or that it's part of nursing or part of teaching but not for presentation in a meeting about psychotherapy. In my view, if a confused and anxious adolescent feels comfortable enough with a particular person to share himself, or parts of himself, then that is an achievement. Disturbed adolescents are so cautious, so afraid; there is a lot of pushing away, of not really trusting anyone. It really matters when someone on the staff has managed to achieve some contact.

I do think it's right for an adolescent unit to have a designated person who offers regular psychotherapy sessions to each boy and girl. But there are the other 166 or 167 hours of the week when adolescents will find their own people to talk to. They need room to feel free to begin to think and talk about themselves, and that may not always be with the designated psychotherapist, at least not in the beginning.

Also, the adolescent's development gains from access to a wide variety of new people; learning from them and finding out different ways of being with them. That is what you would want for all adolescents. And it is part of a good adolescent unit's educational and therapeutic provision.

There are, however, as you say, the dangers of splitting; the tendency in adolescents to place all the good, agreeable, positive aspects of themselves and of their experience in certain people; and dump all the unwanted bits on others. So in that world, the staff are divided into the good and the bad. Now it seems to me that, especially when working with very disturbed adolescents, splitting has to be endured. When you come down to it, it is a primitive, fundamental defensive necessity for some adolescents; they cannot integrate their loving and hating feelings together in relation to the same person. Their very early childhood experiences have not allowed them to; they have never felt safe enough to hate the people they love. They preserve the benign experience with one person; and deposit the hatred and anger onto the other.

What matters is that all the staff are aware of this process; that they are attentive to how an adolescent uses different people. Problems arise when individual staff members get caught up in the adolescent's seductions or denigrations. So that some may feel they have got the knack, that they are only ones who understand the adolescent; and that other staff are too punitive, insensitive, incompetent. Now, this is not to ignore the fact that certain people get along better with some than with others; that not everything in a relationship is a feature of transference. But the tendency of many disturbed adolescents to create split alliances is something to be guarded against. And not least of all in relation to individual psychotherapy. Potentially useful work may be pulled away from formal individual psychotherapy sessions, by another staff member explicitly or implicitly siding with the adolescent's criticism, collecting all the positives for himself or for a group or sub-group of staff, and generally undermining the individual psychotherapy. The converse may occur; the individual psychotherapist riding in a sea of good will, blind to what else is going on and proceeding on the basis that the rest of the staff are having to carry a good deal of hostility and opposition, and perhaps tempted to think with the adolescent that they deserve it.

There are numerous variations on this theme. Rivalries, tensions between staff can be generated or exacerbated. That is why it is so important that there is adequate staff conferencing; to keep some check on these processes and ensure that the adolescent is not caught up in divisions to which in part he has contributed from his own fragmented life.

DS We're talking about understanding what goes on in psychotherapy, and what it does to you. I want to ask you about training; is a personal analysis necessary?

PW I think a personal analysis or therapy is important in most forms of training in individual psychotherapy. It may not produce a perfect human being, but it does at least attend to and mitigate some of the harmful intrusions of psychotherapeutic intervention. And it can increase the capacity to understand another.

DS   It's a hot topic, isn't it, who is competent to be a psychotherapist? I can think of a social worker who took on a patient for regular, supervised psychotherapy, but wanted it to be called casework, not being a trained psychotherapist. Is that correct, or over-conscientious? Again, there are the psychodynamic skills of the nurse–patient relationship. And many psychiatrists who would not describe themselves as psychotherapists practice psychotherapy. Do you think this is an area to be tidied up, regularised?

PW   Clearly different professional groups are based on different disciplines, with different training, emphases, histories. There are distinctive areas of work; ordinarily it happens that they operate separately and similarities and overlap don't matter. But when it comes to joining together in an enterprise such as an inpatient unit, inevitably there will be overlap in practice. And then we are faced with the large question of what is psychotherapy, and who can, or should, practice it. I think there is a danger of getting lost in professional distinctions and elitist pretensions. What matters is being professional about the work; ie. thinking about the therapeutic relationship, trying to understand how the adolescent is using that relationship and what the relationship means for the professional worker; being on the alert for splitting processes, transference, counter-transference. In general, looking critically at what is constituting the helping intervention and what is effective.

DS   What about the distinction between general psychotherapy and specialised psychotherapy that Dennis Brown and Jonathan Pedder make? Is that a useful distinction?

PW   Yes. And I think Brown's and Pedder's book is useful. So too is Garfield's book, and Bloch's. What I think becomes clear is that psychotherapy covers a very broad spectrum of professional activity. What activity takes place depends on a variety of factors: the therapist – his level of experience, his personality, his training and orientation; the adolescent – his developmental state, his psychopathology, his readiness and capacity to seek help; and the interaction between the two. Fundamentally, psychotherapy is a humane and compassionate activity. The essence of it is based on relationship; in individual psychotherapy a relationship between two people. You listen, you care, you bother about some one else. It is basically a process of affirmation and respect for another. Reisman has recognised the many elements that comprise this process and arrived at a brief, broad definition of psychotherapy: 'The communication of person-related understanding, respect and a wish to be of help'. The advantage of such a wide definition is that it takes seriously everything that is going on; that whatever or whoever is concerned, is of potential value. It is a question of knowing what is appropriate, with whom and when.

DS   But what you have said is all rather general. Can you be more specific and distinguish between different kinds of activity? I'm thinking about the components of individual psychotherapy as a treatment, compared with the components of staff-patient relationships which are psychotherapeutic in the more general sense. Is it worthwhile to try to distinguish between what our psychotherapists do and what our nurses, our social workers and our teachers do, for example, in one-to-one relationships with adolescents?

PW   Firstly, I think it helps to think about individual psychotherapy in relation to different kinds of adolescents, with different types of disorder; and then to think about its place in the order of things, as they come to settle around the particular adolescent. It is a question of considering differing needs and sorting out what are the primary goals. Let's break it down into three main levels of activity; the caring, the supportive, the explorative.

To start with, many of the adolescents we see here, particularly in the beginning, are very disorganised. They are confused, lost, disorientated. They have very little sense of themselves, of who they are. Their view of the world is distorted. They are basically terrified, and perceive others dimly, almost as if they don't experience relationships, or they are daunted, expecting attack, indifference or both. They have no basic trust.

These adolescents cannot tolerate or comprehend the closeness or purpose of formal individual psychotherapy sessions. What they need, above all, is people around them who, *in toto*, can provide a setting, an environment of care, nurture and boundary. It is the task of the whole unit to create an atmosphere of care and contact. And the individual therapist takes his place alongside everyone else in achieving that. He may for some time be of less importance to a particular adolescent than other staff members. His sessions may be irregular, often unattended. The individual psychotherapist in that situation has to adapt and extend himself – for example, offering shorter, more frequent sessions, if need be where the adolescent feels safest, not necessarily in the therapy room. He, like everyone else, in one way or another, is trying to get established in the mind of the adolescent; to reach slowly some sort of relationship and trust. That is the primary goal.

DS   Adolescents like these, then, are forming a relationship with the whole unit, or at least a substantial part of it? You would expect that even when we offer a focus of specifically individual psychotherapy for a boy or girl?

PW   The individual psychotherapeutic relationship gradually comes more into focus and significance – as do other relationships – once this early engaging process has taken its course. For some adolescents this may not occur; or it may take a very long time. But if there is some favourable response, progress is possible towards a higher level of psychotherapeutic involvement. The emphasis shifts from something that is fundamentally caring, holding and nurturing, to a more active and effective concern with helping the adolescent to sort out his feelings about himself and others, to get some idea of the effect he has upon others and the realistic and unrealistic ways he sees other people. The psychotherapy is now more about helping the adolescent to make sense of the world, of helping him to contend better with his frustrations and fears and to learn to live more clearly with other people. Some of our adolescents are sufficiently organised to respond to this from the outset.

Again, the individual psychotherapist is but one part of the overall provision of the unit. Other staff members may be actively contributing to this level of psychotherapeutic work; some may focus on behavioural modification, some favour social skills training, others operate cognitive therapy programmes. All, it seems to me, are engaged in a broadly similar level of psychotherapeutic activity – which the psychoanalytically-orientated psychotherapists would call 'ego-strengthening' psychotherapy.

The adolescent himself may at times make more use of other staff members than the designated individual psychotherapist, as we have already said. That is inevitable, and not to be discouraged, provided that what we have said earlier about splitting is taken into account. But, usually, if the individual therapist persists in his relationship with the adolescent, then the chances are that he will increasingly become a particular reference point for the adolescent, and other staff should then encourage this.

DS   I've noticed that you haven't mentioned the word 'interpretation' so far. I must say I discourage interpretation with adolescents. I think it's used too much as a blunt instrument.

PW   No, I think interpretation is important. I think it is an essential part, to complete the job, as it were. But I do think interpretations are often showered about too soon, too frequently, at the wrong time. As if there is a desperate belief that unless interpretation, and particularly interpretation of the transference, is going on, nothing is happening. I hope from what I have said that there can be a whole lot going on besides – caring, containing, facilitating, putting into words, sorting out reality, etc. I don't think that at these levels interpretation has a particularly significant role to play.

For an interpretation to be of any use to an individual it must have two ingredients. Firstly, it must be based on good evidence, ie. it has to be drawn from what that individual himself has communicated to you about himself. Secondly, it must make sense, ie. it must be given in language and in such a way that the individual can hear and understand. Otherwise there is the distinct possibility of the therapist talking in fantasy and leaving the individual mystified. To achieve these two ingredients, the therapist has to establish a relationship with that individual; he has to earn his trust and learn about that individual and how he expresses himself.

Everything that I've just said in general, I believe applies particularly to the disturbed adolescents that we are talking about. You may not be able to get to interpretive work for a long time because the sort of adolescent we see does not feel safe enough; he doesn't know how to be with you; he is so threatened he hardly can hear you; he simply has not reached a position of considering his distress in the light of what you are offering. In other words, you have to create a foundation for interpretation; a foundation based on the elements of care and support that belong to the first two levels of psychotherapy. Once you have established that, you qualify – to know and be heard. There is a greater chance that the adolescent will be talking or communicating more clearly to you; and so you are in a better position to understand and therefore offer interpretation.

DS That's the third level of psychotherapy?

PW Yes. It operates at a higher, more sophisticated level. It's possible with certain adolescents; those who have achieved some greater sense of coherence about themselves; who can see themselves more clearly in relation to others; who have some awareness of how they behave and get along and who don't like the way they are. Their need at this point is for self-understanding; to catch hold of some meaning to their existence, to gain knowledge that will enable them to feel less overwhelmed or buffeted by their feelings. And the goal of psychotherapy at this level is to help facilitate this; to augment insight.

DS This seems to me to be closer to the pure model you were talking about at the beginning. Isn't this what is considered psychotherapy proper? Quite different from what you were describing earlier?

PW I see it as an extension of earlier work, part of an overall process. The difference is a question of emphasis. Interpretation lies at one end of the spectrum of psychotherapeutic intervention. And, from everything that we've said so far, I'm disinclined to call it 'proper'. Proper, in my book, is what is appropriate – appropriate to the needs and the capacities of adolescents, at different developmental levels and with different kinds of psychopathology.

DS I'm interested in your commitment to individual psychotherapy in a unit such as ours. You know what a very mixed group of young people we have here, some not very bright, quite a few with psychotic illnesses. We learn a lot from you when you advise against individual psychotherapy for a particular patient, and hear the reasons why; but more often than not you demonstrate the part psychotherapeutic work plays, whatever the diagnosis, whatever the other treatments. It isn't surprising, perhaps, in the light of the perspective you've described.

PW Well, you see I do have a sort of missionary view about individual psychotherapy. I don't claim its total effectiveness in all cases; nor that it should be applied indiscriminately. But I do see it as a very civilised, humane service offered to another human being. Whatever the diagnosis, however disturbed and chaotic some young people are, one assumes there is some rhyme and reason to their mental lives. Psychotherapy, coming out of psychoanalysis, is essentially to do with meaning; trying to construct some sense about a person's behaviour and thoughts. It is something offered to another person, an opportunity, patiently provided, to find some sort of account of himself. I don't think we know for sure when psychotherapy works, or indeed what 'working' means. But I think that when you get a disturbed human being who is adolescent actually to trust sufficiently to be interested in his own psychological state, and in you, then you are being psychotherapeutic, and achieving something important. As to other treatments, certainly the theoretical differences between certain schools of family therapy and individual therapy do appear to me to be incompatible. We cannot go into these now; much is to do with quite fundamental differences between the intrapsychic and interpersonal viewpoints. As a practitioner, though, I find purity elusive; I'm not pure; and I find incompatibilities not so stubborn. Faced with the extremely difficult problems and mysteries we're presented with here, I'm mostly concerned with what works. But I'm also concerned with the possibility of working at cross purposes, for example conveying paradoxically in a family that a problem is not a problem, or is an insoluble problem; while individually recognising the seriousness of the individual's difficulty and trying hard to help through understanding. I'm not sure we pay enough attention to the effects of different approaches, applied simultaneously, and what the adolescent makes of it all.

You began by asking me what it's like to arrive here to take a consultative session on a Wednesday morning. With great respect to your staff - and I hope you get the drift of the analogy - it's like saying hello to a difficult adolescent patient. I'm pleased to be here - usually; I'm interested and wanting to know. But soon I begin to feel bombarded; flattened, helpless, not a thought in my head. I can only let myself experience the feeling of confusion, risk not knowing, allow anxiety and despair to touch me; and it feels OK to do so. I keep going, listening, thinking, waiting for help, a clue, from within me or outside me, hoping for something new, enlightening, creative to occur between us. Sometimes nothing happens, and the hopelessness hangs about until next time. More often something clicks, and there's a mutual feeling of movement, an accomplishment, a new sense of purpose and meaning and a new way of proceeding. That's why I keep coming; that's why I do psychotherapy.

References and Further Reading

Bloch S (1979) *An Introduction to the Psychotherapies*. New York: Oxford University Press
Brown D & Pedder J (1979) *Introduction to Psychotherapy*. London: Tavistock
Garfield S L (1980) *Psychotherapy: an Eclectic Approach*. New York: Wiley
Kessler E S (1979) Individual Psychotherapy with adolescents. In J R Novello (ed) *The short Course in Adolescent psychiatry*. New York: Brunner/Mazel

Meeks J E (1971) *The Fragile Alliance: an orientation to the Outpatient Psychotherapy of the Adolescent.* Baltimore: Williams & Wilkins

Mueller R L (1977) Self and object in Counter Transference. *International Journal of Psychoanalysis,* **58,** 365–371

Reisman J B (1973) *Principles of Psychotherapy with Children.* New York: Wiley

Wilson P & Hersov L (1984) *Individual and Group Psychotherapy.* In M Rutter & L Hersov (eds) *Child Psychiatry: Modern Approaches.* Oxford: Blackwell

11 The Clinical Psychologist in Adolescent Psychiatry

Derek Bolton

My work in adolescent clinical psychology and psychiatry has been at the Adolescent Unit of the Bethlem Royal and Maudsley Hospitals, which I joined in 1979. My postgraduate training was at the Institute of Psychiatry, associated with the Joint Hospitals. I came into clinical psychology relatively late, my previous work being in philosophical research and writing. In order to qualify for postgraduate training in clinical psychology, one needs a degree in psychology, which I read at University College London.

———◆———

My work as a clinical psychologist divides into several areas. Clinically, I practise various forms of psychological therapy (psychotherapy, behaviour therapy, family therapy), and I am involved in consultation over treatment and management, within and outside the hospital. I also carry out various types of psychological assessment, for example, of cognitive abilities or difficulties. There is a large element of teaching in my work, including the clinical supervision and academic teaching of students on the M Phil course in clinical psychology at the Institute of Psychiatry, and the teaching of nurses and psychiatrists in training. I am engaged also in research and writing. There is no fixed proportion of time given to these different aspects of my work; the amount I spend on each varies from one time to another.

In what follows I shall elaborate on some of these aspects of my work, with emphasis on clinical work within a multidisciplinary team. Where possible, I have tried to generalise about the work of clinical psychologists in hospital adolescent units, but much of what I shall say is specific to me and to the type of institution in which I work; there is much unsaid about the many and varied activities of clinical psychologists in other settings. One aim of the present book is to present personal views, although this, of course, brings with it the disadvantage of partiality. For a comprehensive and detailed description of the development and practice of clinical psychology, the reader is referred to the recent volume edited by Andrée Liddell (1983), and for a thorough account of adolescent services in particular, to the chapter in that volume by Dorothy Fielding (1983).

Psychological Assessment

Much of the clinical psychologist's work in a multidisciplinary team is shared with the members of other disciplines. This applies particularly to the practice of psychological therapies, which will be discussed below. However, there are a number of tasks which are more or less specific to the clinical psychologist, these being concerned mainly with the investigation of cognitive functioning. The most common assessment is of level of intelligence, using the Wechsler Scales for children or adults (WISC or WAIS, or the revised scales, WISC-R and WAIS-R). The purpose of such assessment varies: it may be to assess intelligence at the lower extremes; to investigate learning difficulties, to assess current cognitive function and dysfunction; or as a measure of change over time; and so on. Emphasis in clinical settings is on investigation of the individual case: the I.Q. figure (which relates the individual level to the average level in the population) is relatively less important. Another kind of cognitive assessment concerns the effects of brain damage or dysfunction; for this purpose the so-called 'neuropsychological' tests and procedures are used. The psychologist may also give formal tests of educational attainments (reading, spelling, arithmetic), although these tests would generally be more often used by educationalists (educational psychologists and specialist teachers). Psychologists may also use tests to assess personality traits, though these tend to be used more for research than for clinical purposes.

Psychological assessments of the above kind generally involve other disciplines. Often an assessment responds to a more or less specific question, or series of questions, from a psychiatrist, neurologist, or educationalist. For example: 'To what extent is a child's intellectual performance depressed by a severe emotional disturbance?' or, 'Does a child with known neurological damage have a memory disorder, and of what kind?'; and so on. One type of liaison work needs special mention here, namely, that with educational psychologists in the Schools Psychological Service. The role of the educational psychologist has no separate chapter in this book, which is concerned primarily with hospital inpatient provision, but it may be described briefly and partially here.

Educational psychologists are generally employed by the Education Authorities, and those in the Schools Psychological Service are concerned particularly with psychological problems as they occur in educational settings. One role of the educational psychologist is in the assessment of children with so-called 'special educational needs', ie. needs which perhaps cannot be met within the normal community school provision, and which may therefore require placement at a 'special school'. As part of such an assessment, formal testing of intelligence and educational attainments is advisable, and a clinical psychologist, if already in professional contact with the child in question, may work with an educational psychologist in making this particular part of the assessment. A proportion of adolescents in a psychiatric inpatient unit at any given time are likely to have special educational needs, and may require placement in a special school on discharge, and liaison among these lines.

Another major aspect of work is assessment for treatment. It goes without saying that assessment is required before commencing any form of treatment: assessment of the problem to be worked on, and of indications and contra-indications of therapy. The type of assessment of course depends on the type of therapy being considered. For example, assessment for dynamic psychotherapy usually requires an initial 'in depth' interview; assessment for behaviour therapy includes systematic investigation of the behaviour to be modified, including the use of direct observation.

Psychological Therapies

These include the behaviour therapies and psychodynamic psychotherapy, which are based on more or less well-defined psychological principles, and they are distinguished, in particular, from physically invasive therapies such as pharmacotherapy or electroconvulsive therapy. The practice of these latter therapies belongs exclusively to the medical profession, while the psychological therapies are practised by clinical psychologists, as well as by other mental health professionals (psychiatrists, nurses, social workers, and others).

The range of psychological therapies includes behaviour therapy, dynamic psychotherapy, cognitive therapy, counselling, group therapy, family therapy, psychodrama, and so on, in all their diverse forms. These various forms of treatment are much described in the literature, and some are specifically discussed in this book. The clinical psychologist in a multidisciplinary team would certainly practise one or more forms of psychological therapy. The psychologist would have some freedom in choice of treatment approaches; which one he or she decides to use depends on training, interests and skills, partly on the customs and demands of the institution, as well as on appropriateness for a particular clientele. The so-called eclectic may draw on several approaches according to circumstances, while the specialist will tend to use one type of approach.

The existence of this wide range of psychological therapies, often incompatible among themselves, points to the importance of the idea of a 'body of psychological knowledge', to which controversial topic we turn next.

Psychological Theories and Psychological Science

It might be expected that the scientific or academic study of psychology (as taught in the universities, and as outlined in introductory textbooks) would provide the theoretical background for the work of the clinical psychologist, and indeed partly for the work of the psychiatrist. It is true that scientific psychology has advanced enormously in recent decades, and this has had marked influence on clinical practice. The methods of behaviour therapy, in particular, are now widely used by psychologists and psychiatrists, as in the treatment of excessive anxiety (eg. in school attendance), and in the management of the severely disruptive child. On the other hand, it is debatable how far such methods involve only the laws of conditioning, on which they have usually been said to be based. To cite another kind of example, the rapidly growing field of cognitive psychology has been influential in clinical and educational settings in clarifying the nature of developmental learning difficulties.

The advances made by scientific psychology encourage some clinical psychologists to hold that it provides, or could provide, an adequate basis for clinical practice, but such a view is by no means universally accepted. There is divergence of opinion concerning the nature of the principles underlying the psychological therapies, and the extent to which they are adequately grasped by scientific method. With the growth of scientific psychology, there has been an increasing divide between clinical approaches based on scientific principles (eg. the laws of conditioning), and applying scientific method (such as rigorously objective measures of change), and those approaches based on theories of mind and behaviour which seem, for diverse reasons, less amenable to scientific verification. In brief, and at the risk of oversimplification, there are the behavioural methods and theories on the one hand, and the many and various psychotherapeutic methods, with their associated theories, on the other (for example, psychoanalysis, dynamic psychotherapy, client-centred therapy, transactional analysis, psychodrama, play therapy, systemic family therapy).

The theories behind these psychotherapeutic methods emphasise such concepts as meaning, subjectivity, symbolism and growth, and which by their nature are hard to grasp according to the scientific principles of objectivity, experimentation and generality. But, so the proponents of such theories would say, so much the worse for those principles: science over-reaches itself when it tries to grasp the meaningful life of human beings. On the other hand, again, there is much to be said for the scientific approach in clinical psychology and psychiatry: scientific method aims at knowledge, or at objectively supported hypotheses, and it rejects mere guesswork, indulgent prejudice, or at worst, quack medicine. It seeks results and procedures which can be understood and communicated, rejecting the secrecy of initiation which pervades at least some of the psychotherapies. Thus there exists a tension between on the one hand the demands for scientific rigour and objectivity, and on the other, the spontaneity, complexity and subjectivity of the phenomena encountered in clinical practice. This tension is of practical significance, and I have tried to clarify it from a philosophical point of view in a recent paper (Bolton 1984).

There is a large range of psychological theories which compete as explanations of psychological disorder and of therapy. The divide between scientifically based theories and those which emphasise meaning (the so-called hermeneutical psychologies) is perhaps the most marked, though even within these broad alternatives there are again diverse approaches, for example, as between the theories which draw mainly on learning theory, on cognitive psychology, or on social psychology. The many and various psychological theories, scientific and otherwise, are much described in the literature. It is not my purpose here to list or elaborate them, but merely to point to the fact that there is divergence of opinion as to which theory, or type of theory, is appropriate for clinical work, and hence also no general agreement on how to proceed in practice. Hence the divisions into schools or 'orientations'. And clinical psychologists, like others in the mental health professions, tend to follow one or another, or several, according to their own convictions, and according to the ethos of the institution within which they work.

Psychological Treatment in a Multidisciplinary setting

Enough has been said to indicate that there is no single kind of contribution which clinical psychologists make within a multidisciplinary setting. In general, the psychologist will practise one or more forms of psychological therapy, and indeed he may be the major specialist in such therapy. Conducting psychological therapy in a multidisciplinary setting raises a number of specific issues, mainly concerning the relation between his therapeutic work and the work of others. Where a psychologist is carrying out individual treatment with an inpatient, he needs to keep in close contact with other staff involved; proper communication is essential, to avoid staff working at cross-purposes, and to ensure a constructive consistency of approach. Otherwise much time is wasted, or worse, the client slips untouched between competing policies. Here it may be remarked that the adolescent, particularly one from a disturbed or fragmented family background, is likely to be, at his own expense, a past master at splitting authorities, using one against another, and so on.

This means, in practice, that the psychologist needs to keep other staff adequately informed of the aims, means and progress of therapy. What counts as 'adequate' here needs to be kept under constant review, and is hard to define in advance. Clarification and negotiation are needed particularly if there is, or is likely to be, tension between the psychological therapy and nursing or psychiatric management.

One of the clearest kinds of case under this heading concerns the violent behaviour of one kind or another which may be associated with therapy. Psychotherapy with an adolescent inpatient is likely to be stormy, with potential or actual 'acting out' of this sort, notwithstanding attempts by the therapist to contain violent impulses within sessions, and the adolescent will need a team and unit for containment during the therapy. If this were not necessary, the adolescent would more likely be an outpatient. In this sense the team has responsibility for overall management, of which psychotherapy is one aspect. It is helpful if these issues can be clarified before starting therapy; in that everyone is prepared for the worst. Of course, not all therapeutic approaches give rise to these difficult problems. Others are more gentle, more reliably confined to the therapeutic session itself, and in this case they require rather less team effort. Counselling, supporting psychotherapy, or social skills training would be examples under this heading. On the other hand, probably all psychological therapies may be enhanced by the general therapeutic mileu of the unit. This is connected with the fact that treatment on an inpatient unit can hardly be construed, in general, as happening only in sessions for an hour or two each week. If sessional work were enough, the adolescent would probably be treated as an outpatient. Therapy on an inpatient unit goes on most of the time, in the adolescent's daily living with staff and peers. This 'mileu' therapy includes, for example, encouraging trust, independence, confidence, normal as opposed to symptomatic behaviour, acceptance of appropriate limits, and the development of sound staff and peer relations. Sessional work, psychological treatments of·various kinds, may be necessary to supplement the therapy of the mileu, or in particular, to work on problems which are dealt with insufficiently, or not at all, in the daily routine of the unit; (for example, very poor social skills, severe phobic or obsessional anxiety, or severe problems in intimate personal relations. The clinical psychologist is also likely to be practising family therapy. Family therapy on an in-patient unit raises special issues, which are discussed in another chapter, and which I shall not consider here.

The clinical psychologist carries out treatment directly, but is also likely to have an important role as supervisor or consultant concerning psychological therapies, particularly if he is the team's major specialist in one of these. Apart from acting as supervisor to clinical psychologists in training, the psychologist may also supervise or consult with members of other disciplines, such as nurses or psychiatrists, who are engaged in psychological therapies. Where it is clearly psychological treatment which is in question, the relation between the psychologist and the other disciplines is relatively clear, but the situation is more complex in the vague borderline between psychological treatment and psychiatric or nursing management, where the roles of the respective professionals may not be absolutely clear.

The Role of the Psychologist in the Multidisciplinary Team

The clinical psychologist contributes to the working of a multidisciplinary team in a number of ways already discussed, in assessment, and in treatment, direct or indirect. The psychologist may also contribute particularly to research, whether in treatment trials, or in the experimental investigation of a particular problem, and so on. Research is discussed in a separate chapter, and I shall not elaborate here.

However, the psychologist also contributes something less easy to define, namely, a 'psychological viewpoint' to specific and general management policies. Perhaps this topic can be discussed by considering the strength, as I see it, of a multidisciplinary approach, in an adolescent unit in particular. Each profession brings with it a particular perspective on the adolescent as a whole and on the running of the institution as a whole. I hesitate to summarise these perspectives, which indeed are the subject matter of the present book, but I have in mind the emphasis of psychiatrists on physical health and psychiatric condition, of social workers on relations outside the hospital, of nurses on ward management policies, of teachers and occupational therapists on academic and work education; and so on. The insight which characterises child and adolescent psychiatry in the United Kingdom is that each of these perspectives is necessary if the disturbed adolescent is to be helped to thrive. Nor is this need to pay proper attention to the child as a whole merely a pious ideal; rather it leads to real differences in outcome. It is unsatisfactory if, due to inattention, symptom relief is effected on the ward, but family relations remain so problematic that discharge home is impossible, or likely to result in relapse; or if a withdrawn adolescent's social relations improve, but a potentially incapacitating phobia remains undetected and untreated; or if a psychological treatment is proposed without sufficient regard to what is possible on the ward and in the unit's school; and so forth. Nor is it merely human frailty which makes it difficult for one individual or group to comprehend the many and diverse needs of a disturbed adolescent. For often these needs, and hence the policies which respond to them, may be more or less in conflict with one another, so that catering for one implies playing down another. For example, the approach of a family therapist may well diverge from the individually-orientated policies on the unit, or again, the apparent need of a disturbed adolescent to regress in psychotherapy conflicts with his need also to behave in an age-appropriate way in the unit and at home. These remarks point also to the fact that while a multidisciplinary approach facilitates attention to various aspects of the child's needs, it is absolutely essential that coherent order is made out of them, and that clear policies are made, either by consensus, or by authority.

In this complicated context, the, we may try to define the psychological viewpoint in a multidisciplinary team. Probably above all this viewpoint would depend on the orientation of the individual psychologist (eg. behavioural or psychodynamic). Considering further what the several psychological orientations have in common, for the present purpose, the psychologist would tend to view disturbance not in psychiatric terms (eg. not primarily in terms of psychiatric diagnosis, or of illness), but in such terms as maladaptive learning, traumatic experience, or deficiency in skills or coping strategies. Given formulation in such terms, the psychologist would aim to encourage the development of new patterns of interpretation and behaviour. This may involve partly psychological treatment, but clearly it involves also general management policies, particularly on the ward.

This leads on to the role of the psychologist in contributing to ward management policies. As mentioned in the previous section, the role of the psychologist is relatively clear insofar as one can define a treatment as a clearly psychological therapy, perhaps involving behavioural principles, such as social skills training, desensitization of phobias, response-prevention for obsessive-compulsions, or a token-economy programme. But the relation of psychologist to nursing team is less clear in the grey area between psychological therapy and nursing management policy. In formulating management policy, and in spontaneous response to events as they happen, the nursing team sets limits, draws out the withdrawn child, and generally encourages appropriate behaviour, all of which is closely connected to psychological principles and practice, and which may in a particular case be a major aspects of treatment. For this reason the psychologist may consult with the nursing team, or with senior nurses, over management policies. Such consultation needs careful handling on both sides. At worst, the risk is that neither side feels valued by the other. This seems to happen particularly when both parties collude in the view that the psychologist is trying to do (or is being asked to do) nursing work at a distance, without understanding nursing work, and most of all without having to undertake it directly. It is better when each can acknowledge the particular skills and experience of the other: the psychologist's therapeutic skills in application to management, and the nurses' skills in the management of a ward full of very disturbed adolescents. Within this context consultation between psychologist and nursing team is necessary and may be very effective.

I turn now to the relation of the psychologist to other professional groups in a multidisciplinary team, particularly social workers and psychiatrists. Psychologist and social worker have in common that they are non-medical, and likely to specialise in forms of psychological therapy. Relations between them are in these respects close, particularly insofar as they have the same or similar clinical orientation. Psychologists and psychiatrists have in common a dominant concern with treatment issues, including the use of psychological therapies. However, the relation between psychologist and psychiatrist is conditioned by a number of structural factors, the main one being that the consultant psychiatrist always has medical responsibility for inpatients, and hence for the psychologist's work with them. In this sense the psychologist is answerable to the psychiatrist, as well as to his own profession. This means that the relationship between psychiatrist and psychologist can be broadly of two types. In one, the psychiatrist may wish to be highly involved in the psychologist's work, to the extent of making it difficult for the psychologist to function freely and effectively as therapist. This causes problems which need to be resolved. In the other, and better, the psychiatrist allows autonomy to the psychologist, obviously within the limits of his judgement as to the patient's wellbeing. There are in general a number of formal parameters which partly define the relations between the various mental health professions, but within these parameters there is scope for a wide variety of possibilities, depending on individual and institutional temperaments. It is hard to generalise about these important and influential informal relationships and institutional patterns. So far as concerns the clinical psychologist in the structure of a multidisciplinary team, one of the most important and common features is that he or she will have a natural seniority in matters of psychological treatment and management, deriving from scientific training, from an understanding of psychological principles, and from experience as a therapist.

References and Further Reading

Bolton D (1984) Philosophy and psychiatry. In P McGuffin, M Shanks & R Hodgson (eds) *Scientific Principles of Psychopathology*. London: Academic Press

Bolton D & Turner T (1984) Obsessive-compulsive neurosis with conduct disorder in adolescence: a report of two cases. *Journal of Child Psychology and Psychiatry*, **25**, 133–139.

Fielding D (1983) 'Adolescent Services'. In A Liddell (ed) *The Practice of Clinical Psychology in Great Britain*. Chichester: Wiley

Liddell A (1983) *The Practice of Clinical Psychology in Great Britain*. Chichester: Wiley

12 The Psychiatrist and the Adolescent Unit

Derek Steinberg

I trained in medicine at the London Hospital and in psychiatry at Brookwood Hospital, the National Hospitals for Nervous Diseases at Queen Square and Maida Vale, the Maudsley, and the Park Hospital for Children, Oxford. In 1973 I was appointed consultant psychiatrist at the regional adolescent unit, Long Grove Hospital, and soon after began the Tavistock Clinic's training in consultation and community mental health. In 1975 I was appointed consultant at the Adolescent Unit and Children's Department at Bethlem Royal Hospital and the Maudsley. Other professional activities related to the theme of this book include being a clinical advisor and examiner on the Goldsmiths' College Art Therapy Course, taking a fortnightly staff training group at Adelaide House Children's Home in North Kensington, and teaching at the University of Surrey, now as honorary visiting Reader in psychiatry and human development. I am also involved in the Maudsley Hospital's Staff Working Groups training programme.

———◆———

The week's work consists of meetings. Not for the most part committee meetings, fortunately, but meetings with patients; meetings with families; meetings with unit staff working with patients and families; and meetings with colleagues in the hospital and elsewhere about matters which affect the operation of the unit. Many of these meetings are informal, for example with a boy or girl in the lounge or the pottery room; others planned, for example, when I meet the adolescent with his registrar, or meet child and family with several members of staff to review progress.

The week has its fixed points. There is the new referral meeting when we hear about young people referred to the unit in the last few days and discuss how best to respond; the 'routine' new patient assessment – routine perhaps for us, anything but routine for the adolescent and family; the ward round, when we look at the progress and objectives we minuted last time, and the subsequent developments; the meetings which in various ways look in more depth at work in progress, for example Christopher Dare's family therapy consultation session, Peter Wilson's individual psychotherapy consultation, small-group supervision which I take with Teresa Wilkinson, and a monthly review of outpatient work. We distinguish between supervision (by the staff members' formal seniors who are responsible for their teaching and share responsibility for their work) and consultation (provided by a specialist, but with formal responsibility remaining with staff members and seniors). This is one way of widening the experience of all of us without causing confusion about who is in charge of a particular piece of work. Another contribution to the range of teaching and treatment is the fact that three other consultants (Michael Rutter, Eric Taylor and Phillip Connell) have inpatients on the unit and take ward rounds. This arrangement works because we have managed to distinguish between general management issues (where I represent the medical point of view) and individual treatment issues (the responsibility of the consultant in charge of the patient's case).

There are, of course, additional events, some unscheduled, some best described as complicated. This week we have had an emergency meeting with a social work office and its lawyer about an inpatient whisked home by the solitary, troubled parent, incommunicado and perhaps at risk; an interview with 16-year-old transexual, sometimes suicidal adolescent, the family and the staff about which pronoun (he or she) and which showers (boys or girls) to use on admission, with the staff very conscious of that fine balance between ethics, respect for individual choice and a need for consistent authority if we are to see a stormy admission through in a therapeutic way. We have visited a children's home to see a highly-dependent 15-year-old, largely mute and so immobile that her hands and feet go blue; a meeting with the hospital administration and lawyers and the three inpatient units (the children's unit, ourselves and the unit for mental handicap) about our right, if any, to detain young people even briefly if they are not on sections of the Mental Health Act; a visit by a Health Advisory Service Team; and by some fire prevention officers, followed shortly after by a small fire, and the subsequent temporary absconding of the offender who claimed, wrongly, that we had reacted too strictly. Those familiar with adolescent units will recognise a fairly characteristic sample of events.

What are medical practitioners contributing in this field?

Medicine

Until fairly recently (and still, in some quarters) the second oldest profession was regarded as a special source of parental and often paternal wisdom in the community, along with the Church and the Law. Even now, when engineers and economists with PhDs pronounce on public issues they may well find newspaper headline writers awarding gratuitous medical accolades, as if that set the seal of authority: 'Dr X's prescription', or 'Dr Y's bitter pill'. For whatever reason, partly historical and partly cultural, physicians have always claimed an interest in the human condition and the human psyche as well as the body, and have tended to encourage exploration of the relationships between all three. This medical-social duality has been useful, because we have often seen progress in clinical and scientific aspects of medicine translated into social policy and public education before real progress in public health has been possible. The control of malnutrition and infection are two examples, and lung cancer and heart disease may prove to be two more. The relationship between clinical progress in psychiatry and public policy is a more complex matter.

Medicine is Janus-faced in another, more curious sense, too, on the one hand sober and scientific, on the other associated in the public mind with frivolity and worse. Perhaps this is understandable, and necessary, considering the tasks Medicine undertakes. This permission for diversity has impact on the practice of medicine which delves with enthusiasm into every conceivable field, and from which, every so often, individual doctors 'break out' into poetry, politics and – a notable sub-specialty – television comedy. There is no doubt that the spirited adventurism of the medical profession offends some whose disciplines are more tightly run in terms of role, training, rules and so on. Professional diversity does have its dark side, and it isn't surprising that *Roget's Thesaurus* lists under the heading 'Jack of all trades' not only the entry *proficient person* but *bungler* too. It has its more sinister aspect, too, in the oppressive, interfering aspects of medical intervention stated or overstated by Szasz (1961) amongst many others, and with more sophistication by Foucault (eg. Foucault 1967; Sheridan 1980). Yet Foucault, while drawing attention to the way in which Medicine, with its prison-like buildings and approaches, took over the care of the insane from the monasteries (and Bethlem, of course, began as a monastery), says also that we must acknowledge, for example, the contribution of Freud who 'did not make a major addition to the list of psychological treatments for madness (but) restored, in medical thought, the possibility of a dialogue with unreason', (Foucault 1967). The academic neurologist Freud developed psychoanalysis, and it has been psychiatrists who pioneered the psychotherapies, psychodrama, art therapy, special education, the therapeutic community, family therapy and even the 'antipsychiatry' movement, as well as the institutional and biological aspects of psychiatry.

Doctors are helped as innovators by two things: a wide social, biological and cultural perspective, and a social status which permits us, up to a point, to take risks with resources and with people. There is no doubt that progress in organisational policies and in clinical practice can be hazardous. The peculiar status of Medicine, generally positive but always ambivalent, has helped psychiatry, the professions associated with it, and its patients, too, by lending all a degree of respectability (earned by more established doctors and scientists) while our proper clinical, scientific and ethical credentials and the seriousness of the subject have gradually become established.

Psychiatry

There are very many ways of being a psychiatrist in adolescent psychiatry, and if one examines them all the impression is of a broad and variegated specialty, not a narrow one. It is possible to be primarily a family therapist, or a developer of therapeutic communities, or to take a special interest in neurodevelopmental disorders and mental handicap, for example. Probably it is fair to divide the field into the psychotherapists and the general psychiatrists, those in each camp not really convinced that those in the other can be both.

The details of different psychiatrists' practice is likely to vary. Many will do some consultative work and varying amounts of teaching and research, depending on opportunity as well as aptitude and interest. Most, perhaps, would be prepared to prescribe medication for some adolescents, but this too is likely to be variable; psychiatrists are likely to choose work which matches their interests and this will include their willingness to see adolescents with disorders that respond to drugs. About a third of my inpatients are on medication (see Chapter 21) *because* I and my colleagues emphasise psychotherapeutic, family therapeutic and consultative approaches to keep young people out of hospital, with some success; those who cannot be held in the community in this way, and are admitted, tend to include a large minority with disorders which need medication. These young people also need a therapeutic setting, family work and in some cases psychotherapy, and it would be unfortunate if adolescent psychiatric units evolved in such a way that young people would receive either medication, or psychotherapy, but not both in the same place. Medication, however, is a subject that tends to polarise people, and there is some evidence that it could become a declining interest among entrants to child psychiatry (Garralda 1980), even though it is one of the few skills special to doctors.

What else can we do that no-one else can do? The question is worth asking because we are fairly expensive. Firstly, most psychiatrists seem to retain a clinical 'feel' for physical disorder even when general medical experience is far behind. What is important is not so much the rare discovery of a cerebral tumour or metabolic disease, but a general familiarity with healthy and unhealthy physical development. It enables us to balance risks when, for example, treating anorexia nervosa, or to know how best to respond to headaches and bellyaches in a particular adolescent's case; and, like general practitioners, when to call in the specialist. It also enables us to talk the same language as other doctors, for example in general practice, community health, paediatrics and neurology. This obviously helps us, our non-medical colleagues and our patients, but also enables psychological and psychiatric thinking to inform general medical care.

We can sign sections of the Mental Health Act, although there is a limit to how much we can do by ourselves, and we can act as free agents in clinical work, taking on and admitting patients. This autonomy at consultant level, quite divorced from any administrative or supervisory hierarchy, is not unique to doctors but is very nearly so (Black & Harris 1978). Psychologists in hospitals may increasingly be able to work autonomously, but most other professions are answerable to senior colleagues. I would like to see others, particularly senior nurses, share the position consultants have, where no further move away from work with patients is necessary unless the practitioner particularly desires it (although there may be some who would prefer to see consultants within the restraints of an 'outside' hierarchy).

We are also interested in the patient's individual mental state, something sometimes underplayed in child and adolescent psychiatry because we see so many young people who are clearly responding normally to anomalous family and social circumstances. Nevertheless, it is important, and probably even family and individual psychotherapists (those who are trained as psychiatrists) have and use a sense of the referred patient's mental state, without having to side-track to formal individual examination unless they conclude it is really necessary. The point is often made by family therapists that family assessment can proceed to individual work, if necessary, but that the reverse is not so easy (Dare 1985). Some adolescent services – I do not know how many, or how they are distributed – will only see the family, and not make time to see the individual boy or girl as well. The work of Leff and his colleagues (Leff & Vaughn 1981; Leff *et al* 1982) and Bolton *et al* (1983) are only two examples of developments in treatment which depend on acknowledgement of both individual *and* family factors. It is easy, it seems, for practitioners in all disciplines to slip into the belief that one aspect of people's lives is the 'real' cause of problems, other factors being subsidiary by some trick of nature or social circumstances. I think it is a contribution of the medical approach that individual factors continue to be regarded as important in assessment and treatment, despite social changes or 'advances'; and that these factors may be psychodynamic, psychobiological or psychosocial, but still the concern of the individual, who has a right to individual attention and to employ his or her individual practitioner, medical or otherwise.

This willingness to draw upon a whole range of conceptual models to try to make sense of psychiatric problems is central to the medical approach (Clare 1982; Tyrer & Steinberg 1986). Some models may be incompatible with each other (eg. some social *versus* individual notions of aetiology) but this does not make them invalid, because we can hardly know which factors are operating with which relative weights in individual patients.

All this could be read as a simplistic argument for the 'medical model' being best, but this is not the case, or at least not the argument. The individual doctor will not be skilled enough in many or most of the areas he or she sees as important in aetiology, assessment or treatment, and this is undoubtedly true in child and adolescent psychiatry. He or she will want, and need, to work with experts in these other areas; but will often want, or need, to have the last word when there is disagreement about the patients' care, or at least to be able to decide when to allow others the last word. The basis for this medical view is twofold: firstly, that the patient is entitled to have a doctor who takes ultimate professional responsibility, and secondly, that in the end, in a field so full of ambiguities and uncertainties of every sort, only one person's clinical judgement can prevail, until the patient (and family) seeks that of someone else. This latter point is no small one. The patient and family have an informal contract with a doctor, not with a hospital, a department or a 'service', and their right to that personal arrangement deserves preservation despite doctors' need for collaboration with other professions, other agencies and with less personal hierarchies. There are, after all, other doctors, other professionals, and other models of care. The medical approach is not therefore the unopposed 'best', but it has clear characteristics which can be accepted or rejected (by the clientele). It also contains inevitably the seeds of dispute with other professional workers, and the tension that results can be creative or dissipating.

The Psychiatrist's Role in the Adolescent Unit

Stated at its simplest, I see the primary responsibility of the psychiatrist as ensuring that each adolescent is well enough, mentally and physically, to take part in a ward and school milieu which is educational, therapeutic and enjoyable. The aim of this exercise is to enable the boy or girl to return to a more natural setting where much the same can be provided less clinically, as quickly as makes sense. When that means treating symptoms and checking mental state, physical health and medication, while others undertake art therapy, family therapy, psychotherapy and fun and games, as it sometimes does, then that is a respectable enough function for a psychiatrist.

Of course, it is not that simple, because psychiatrists on the unit take part in all these other things too, but I believe it important for each profession to take authority and responsibility for its core functions and contribution. Doing so, as mentioned in Chapter 21, helps rather than hinders crossing professional boundaries. Having made clear that anybody may do practically anything, if trained or supervised, (and in practice they do), it is worth outlining some of the equivalent primary contributions of other disciplines, as they seem to a psychiatrist.

The nurses do the nurturing (nourishing, fostering, rearing, training), from which the name of the profession comes. They hold the patients and hold the unit together round the clock while the other clinical professionals tend to work more sessionally. They provide a material basis for work: food, drink, warmth and safety, as well as nursing and treatment. While the psychotherapist or family therapist is seeing the patient, for example, the charge nurse is arranging the patient's tea. The patient goes back to the ward from his session, perhaps puzzled and troubled by it, and has a cup of tea with a nurse, who lets him talk it over, while keeping the boundaries of the therapeutic session and the chat over tea quite clear. In this and innumerable other ways I see the nursing staff as maintaining other people's therapies as well as those they do themselves. Somehow they do this, and meet parents at visits and weekends, without undermining the work of those who work with parents; or the parents themselves.

The teachers in our school look after the other side of the 'milieu', and provide what is the most natural, normal component of it. As with all good schools the activities are creative and fun as well as academic and remedial. It is an excellent thing to see parents and children coming to parents' evenings in the school, looking for all the world like ordinary people, which they do not quite seem in the video studio or through the one-way screen. The school is a constant reminder and reinforcer of everyone's normal, non-clinical, less-institutional side.

Occupational therapists seem also to have this happy aptitude for encouraging the natural and the normal, with the emphasis on occupational and leisure skills as the means or as the end. Just as the teachers link us and the adolescents with outside schools, past and future, occupational therapists make connections with further training and with future work.

Social workers take the lead in family therapy and family work and help with the supervision of both. They maintain liaison with workers in the community over information-gathering and in planning discharge, and sustain social links between the adolescent and the outside world, not only through family and extended family, but by helping to remind us of legal, ethical and cultural requirements of children and families from the most varied backgrounds and circumstances. This affirmation of other people's rights and wishes is not always easy or straightforward; we have had girls from families who discouraged attendance at the unit's discos or contact with boys, for example, quite punitively some of us thought. Our social workers tend to stand up for the parents' views as those which they are entitled to hold, however 'non-therapeutic' they seem to be.

Our psychologist is a psychotherapist, behaviour therapist and family therapist as well as a scientist; it is as someone who can also translate questions about assessment, treatment and the monitoring of treatment into something objective and measurable that his full contribution is particularly recognised. Over the years the unit's senior psychologists have acted first as teachers, then as consultants, particularly to the nursing staff, in this respect. They help us to clarify the possibilities and limitations of psychological science.

These colleagues are present at the ward round and on the other occasions when we review progress and make management plans. Together they provide a composite picture of what the boy or girl is like, of what is working and what is not working, and of what might work. It enormously widens the psychiatrists' perceptions from what the adolescent said to what he or she actually does, in different circumstances, with different people, around the clock. I see an important part of my own role in trying to co-ordinate this professional activity for the unit, weaving various threads together and directing, influencing, consulting about, teaching, learning or turning a blind eye, whichever seems right. The purpose, for me, is that stated above: to see what we can all do to help the adolescent function at his best, and to make constructive use of the milieu, which means the people in it; and to move back or on to more natural and more appropriate friendships, relationships and responsibilities as soon as possible.

People not present at clinical meetings tie threads together in other ways. Two of the several fixed points which permit elasticity are represented by the secretaries and by the staff group. Secretaries put things down on paper, among other activities, which discourages prevarication: this is what we decided to do, who it will involve, and when and where we will meet. They record the work we do. The staff group picks up what's left over when action and decisions have been taken: good feelings, bad feelings and muddled feelings, from which we all can learn something for next time.

My own attention to the individual adolescent, and his experience of the unit, clearly straddles individual diagnosis and treatment on the one hand and the management of the milieu as a whole on the other. It also involves what the boy or girl is going on to, at home or in a new home. A careful balance has to be achieved if all of us directly involved with an adolescent's case – clinical psychiatrist, family therapist, nurse, and social worker, for example – are to make the most of each other's skills in the interests of the patient. A static balance can be achieved by direction, but the dynamic balance needed in eclectic treatment requires everyone to take some responsibility for equilibrium; it sometimes requires acrobatics too, and very occasionally, prestidigitation.

I certainly see the psychiatric contribution as something of a balancing, and counterbalancing, performance. It is not only to do with selecting from the range of conceptual models referred to earlier; it also concerns recognition that biological, psychological and social perspectives have become separated for academic and administrative purposes, not because people actually function according to compartmentalised rules. Everything that we know about the development and functioning of young people points to the necessity to understand the interaction between chemistry, neurology, perceptions, feelings and culture if we are to help where ordinary, common sense approaches do not work – which, it seems to me, is where psychiatry becomes useful. On the one hand this approach could be criticised as too all-embracing, too uncertain, too much concerned with *ad hoc* , pragmatic remedies; but it is a powerful antidote to single-perspective, single-solution approaches, whose proponents seem sometimes to follow Ruskin's dictum about how to establish what is good: 'you assert without vacillating'. I appreciate, and use with gratitude, the confidence and competence of therapeutically specialised colleagues, but *I* know that *they* do not know why one patient responds to medication plus education, another to small group work and a youth training scheme, another to family therapy and counselling by a nurse. I find many of my patients baffling, and am thankful for the medical perspective, part science and part art, which helps me ask questions which seem to lie primarily within biology and anthropology, and appropriately so.

This short account has not discussed teaching and research, which should be a contribution made by all disciplines. Psychiatrists (and psychologists) tend to be the only professionals *expected* to undertake research and encourage others to do so too. Of course, we should encourage systematic studies, but we need also to remind our colleagues how little we know about the nature of the problems which come our way, or what will significantly help, so that questions and doubts are regarded as every bit as important as the assertion of authority. Finding questions that can be answered is the first step in scientific enquiry. However, we need also live with questions that cannot be answered, those aspects of people's lives for which science and clinical technology will remain inadequate. Perhaps doctors, reliant on art as well as science, have a contribution to make here too.

References and Further Reading

Black M & Harris J (1978) 'From 'child guidance' to 'child and family psychiatry': problems of interdisciplinary communication

Bolton D, Collins S & Steinberg D (1983) The treatment of obsessive–compulsive disorder in adolescence. *British Journal of Psychiatry*, **142**, 456–464

Clare A (1982) In M Shepherd (ed) Psychiatrists on Psychiatry. Cambridge University Press

Foucault M (1967) *Madness and Civilisation*. London: Tavistock

Garralda H M E (1980) Trainee s'attitudes in child psychiatry. *Bulletin of the Royal College of Psychiatrists*, February, 26–27

Leff J P & Vaughn C E (1981) The role of maintenance therapy and relatives' expressed emotion in relapse of schizophrenia: a 2-year follow-up. *British Medical Journal*, **139**, 102–104

Leff J P, Kuipers L, Berkowitz R, Erberlein-Vries R & Sturgeon D (1982) A controlled trial of social intervention in the families of schizophrenic patients. *British Journal of Psychiatry*, **141**, 121–134

Rowbottom R & Bromley G (1976) *Future Organisation in Child Guidance and Allied Work*. Institute of Organisation and Social Studies, Brunel University, London

Royal College of Psychiatrists (1978) The role, responsibilities and work of the child and adolescent psychiatrist. *Bulletin of the Royal College of Psychiatrists*, July, 127–131

Sheridan A (1980) *Michel Foucault*. London: Tavistock

Steinberg D, Tyrer P (1986) *Models for Mental Disorder*. Chichester: Wiley, in press

Szasz T (1961) *The Myth of Mental Illness*. New York: Hoeber-Harper

The Adolescent Unit
Edited by Derek Steinberg
© 1986 D. Steinberg

13 The Secretary

Jean Winship

I trained as a junior medical secretary, and after various posts in general hospitals in the NHS came to live in London and then to work on the Adolescent Unit at Bethlem Royal Hospital in 1968. Since 1976 the Unit's outpatient and community work has developed considerably, and there is now closer involvement with the Children's Department at the Maudsley Hospital. Additional secretaries have been employed to cope with the work generated by this expansion and there are now more medical, social work, psychology, teaching and nursing staff on the Unit than in 1968, an increase that includes a greater number of temporarily-attached trainees in all disciplines, which also means a higher frequency of changes among the staff.

I am now employed as senior secretary on the Unit and personal secretary to the consultant in administrative charge. Over the years the secretarial duties have become more complex, the administrative and organisational aspects of my work becoming more prominent. As senior secretary I am involved in planning and staff meetings and expected to contribute to discussions concerning administrative issues of all degrees of importance, responsibilities that go well beyond the usual basic secretarial duties of typing and passing on messages. Being given the opportunity and encouragement to make a contribution in this way has been personally rewarding and I believe has made the administration of the Unit's team more efficient and effective. I believe that similar teams could benefit if suitably-trained and experienced secretaries were able to work in the same way.

———•———

The Adolescent Unit's 'production' includes patients in all degrees of recovery, some relieved parents, many interested visitors (300–400 in 1983), a large number of staff in training (some 60–70 each year), and vast quantities of paper – letters, summaries, reports, appointments, waiting lists, memos, messages, announcements and all the documentation that inpatients, outpatients and day patients require. This traffic in people and pieces of paper, supplemented by telephone calls in and out all through the day is handled by the unit secretaries; it represents not only information to be conveyed but also to an extent reflects some of the feelings of the staff, of the adolescents and their families and of professional workers from outside the Unit. All this has necessitated administrative procedures and systems being set up and maintained and makes a number of quite complex demands of the secretary.

First and foremost, there is a need for sympathy with and understanding of the team's philosophy and its work with adolescents, their families and their problems.

Secretaries attend new referral meetings, outpatient supervision meetings, business meetings, staff groups and our six-monthly staff training days. This helps them get the 'feel' of how the Unit operates. It not only helps in administration but in the style of one's response to patients, families, professional workers and, not least, new staff.

The administrative area of the Unit is a group of 14 rooms linked directly with the wards which are the living and sleeping areas for the boys and girls, seven days a week. Only very occasionally is the ward area 'closed off', and any secretary working on the Unit expects contact with 'disturbed' boys and girls. She must be able to work in an environment that can include lots of noise, pop music, shouting, laughter, crying, screaming. She must be able to cope with interruptions and the busy comings and goings of the members of the entire team. Noisy, intrusive boys and girls, although told that the office area is out of bounds nonetheless find their way into the reception area and can make nuisances of themselves. Sometimes the secretary has to observe the demarcation lines and ring for a nurse to take the adolescent back to his proper activity. Yet it is also necessary to know how to respond to a friendly, naturally inquisitive gesture. With nurses and secretaries seeing each other on a daily basis, it is possible to know in advance what is an appropriate action to take with individual boys and girls. For example, it would be inappropriate to approach a boy or girl, behaving badly, who was known to react violently – far better for the secretary to leave the young person alone and quietly and discreetly ring for a nurse. Equally, to respond too coolly to an inhibited child would be a missed opportunity.

Knowing how to respond effectively and appropriately to outside callers is an essential skill for a secretary working in a hospital setting. Frantic telephone calls from outside agencies, desperate to 'place' adolescents or in a hurry for information, come via the secretary. It is sometimes impossible for the appropriate doctor or social worker to be available to answer and deal with such calls with the immediacy that may be expected. The secretary can help, being familiar with the broad lines of the Unit's policy for admissions, the current bed-state, and waiting list, and knowing when someone will be able to ring the caller back and to whom to pass on messages. This helps the enquirer and can save valuable time for the caller and the members of the clinical team.

Secretaries receive telephone calls from parents, too, asking to speak to someone, often sounding anxious and upset. She will need to be able to know how to judge the request and sense when interrupting members of staff in their work is necessary. Knowing something of the parents, the child and the background is a help in determining how best to respond, and this is guided by the secretary's knowledge of the broad lines along which her colleagues work. Often, letting parents know that their messages will be passed on as soon as possible and that you can understand their anxiety, is sufficient to help them wait for a little while.

Over the years the Unit has placed considerable emphasis on the way in which it receives newcomers, whether boys and girls, their families, visitors or new staff. This represents a very large number of people each day, and the secretary is very often the first person the newcomers will meet. The secretaries will of course want to be friendly, smiling, and relaxed; in the circumstances this can be more easily said than done. We like to have coffee available, too, when some of the families travel from a distance. We also try to ensure that the waiting area is reasonably pleasant, and that those waiting are not liable to overhear other people's conversations. We take some preliminary details of new patients and register their attendance at the hospital. It is important to be aware how anxious parents and children can be about attending a 'mental hospital', especially if it is for the first time. What is rewarding is the occasional comment 'What a nice place', or 'It's better than we thought it would be'.

At the moment we have two dogs on the staff as well; we have had three. They belong to the secretaries, and their involvement in reception produces visible signs of relaxation in many parents and children. But we must always be aware how mixed the feelings of parents and children can be, and there can be a good deal of tension, anger and embarrassment, too. Dealing in a confident, friendly but non-intrusive way with families, and judging what will help, is quite a challenge.

As part of a teaching hospital, the Adolescent Unit has a high turnover of staff in training, about which we, too, can have mixed feelings. The secretary makes a conscious effort to try to make new staff welcome, and it has been found helpful to give beginners handouts in the form of a summary of their duties, a list of telephone numbers and staff on the Unit, timetables, a news-sheet and other such documents. Much time is spent in explaining how the Unit works, and a proportion of staff will, of course, be new to the whole Hospital and Institute. Its administrative systems, who's who, simple day-to-day matters such as knowing where the offices are, where to get keys, tea and coffee, times of hospital transport, what time the canteen opens and shuts – all this is an essential part of making staff feel welcome and helping them to fit in.

Permanent staff have to expect that newcomers will bring with them different ideas of how to do things, and secretaries can equally expect to hear of brilliant new proposals. If the idea is a good one, it will be tried out and perhaps incorporated, but at times it is necessary to state firmly but politely that certain systems have been running smoothly and efficiently for several years and that the intention is for them to continue to do so.

Liaison and communication is demanding. At the Adolescent Unit the secretary is involved in the documentation and recording of every referral that comes through to the team, whether or not the referral actually becomes a patient of the Unit. The number of referrals and enquiries to the Unit numbers some 300–400 every year. At times there can be a large number of different professionals involved in the overall management of each child and family, and supervision of the work. It is important that the secretary should know to whom to communicate information, whether about a new referral or enquiry or about a current patient. A large office diary is used by the doctors, social workers, psychologists and senior nurses to record their whereabouts, their appointments, family meetings, and so on (or it should!). This simple system is a method for knowing when staff will be available to respond to enquiries, it helps in documenting the numbers of patients and visitors seen during the month, and helps in the allocation of rooms for teaching sessions, family meetings, and so on. A weekly News-sheet, issued in place of memos, timetables and announcements, has proved helpful; it has aided the process of looking and planning ahead, and helped co-ordination so that with the secretary's help clashes of time and place are avoided. The News-sheet contains 'news' as well as reminders about formal meetings.

```
                      ADOLESCENT UNIT - NEWSHEET
                 Notes for week commencing 30 January 1984


 MONDAY 30.1.84                      THURSDAY 2.2.84
 Management meeting -Downstairs      Ward Round  Dr Taylor's Patients 9.30 am
   Conference Room 9.30 am                       Dr Steinberg's Patients 10.45 am
 TUESDAY 31.1.84                                 (Outside SW attending 11.30 am - patient DT)
 New assessment-Patient AF (Dr.Thiels/       Family Therapy Consultation - Edward Cooper Unit 12.30 pm
   Lynette Hughes SW/Pete Short TE1)          Community group 4.15 pm
   Outside SW attending case discussion  FRIDAY 3.2.84
   11-15 am                           Staff Group - Downstairs Conference Room 10 am
 Community group 4.15 pm              New Referrals Meeting- Upstairs Conference Room  11.15 am
 Evening activity for children - ice skating  Senior Staff Group - Upstairs Conference Room 12.15 pm
 WEDNESDAY 1.2.84
 Unit Planning Meeting - Upstairs Conference
   Room. 9.15 am
 Psychotherapy Consultation - Downstairs
   Conference Room 10.30 am
                       Dates for Diaries-
             Tuesday 6.2.84 Outpatient Supervision Meeting - agenda to be circulated
             Wednesday 7.2.84 Visitors' Day. Organisers - Alison and Gary
             Friday 10.2.84 Farewell drink for Lucy 5.30 pm onwards at The Wheatsheaf. All staff welcome
                        . . . . . . . . .
             On leave  Adrian Angold away 30.1.84 back 6.2.84
                       Derek Bolton  away 30.1.84 back 6.2.84
                       Bill Payne  away 1.2.84 back 10.2.84
                        . . . . . . . . .
             NB Seminars on Consultation - 3 sessions beginning 8.2.84.See Celia for details
```

New referrals' details and enquiries for advice are taken by staff throughout the seven-day week, collected by the senior registrar and the secretary and discussed at the weekly Referrals Meeting. Urgent matters, dealt with at the time of the enquiry, are mentioned at the meeting and the action taken is recorded. After discussion some referrals will be given a date for an appointment for assessment and the psychiatric registrar, social worker and a nurse from one of the wards will be allocated the child's case and initiate assessment plans. One of our senior teachers joins the referral meeting and often plays a part in the child's assessment. The secretary is at this meeting and takes the minutes, recording the range of decisions: any appointments made, advice or information given, a meeting to be arranged to get further details or to clarify a referral, consultative work set up, an admission date fixed, or sometimes simply 'no further action'.

An agenda for the ward rounds, held on Thursdays, is prepared by the senior registrar. He does this at the Management Meeting on a Monday morning when all the boys and girls are briefly reviewed and dates fixed for a fuller discussion, to which outside professional workers may be invited. With four consultants having beds in the Unit and the large numbers of staff involved, this can be a complex business, and more so when urgent situations arise and necessitate a change of agenda.

Following the ward round, the registrars prepare a brief management decisions document on their patients. This is typed, recorded in the notes and distributed to other key members of staff involved in the treatment of the children.

The Unit Planning Meeting, held every six weeks, is the business meeting of the Unit, attended by senior staff and chaired by the consultant. It is concerned with the long-term planning as well as the administration and day-to-day running of the establishment as a whole. The secretary attends this meeting as a senior member of staff, and is expected to make a contribution to administrative issues that arise or are likely to arise in the light of forthcoming developments. For example, visitors days; forthcoming teaching and study days; changes of policies on the Unit and within the Hospital; trades union matters; confidentiality; legal and ethical aspects in the care of patients, both our own concerns and those arising from outside. The Unit is part of a most complex network of agencies and employers: the Department of Health and Social Security, the Inner London Education Authority, the local Department of Social Services and the Institute of Psychiatry of the University of London, as well as being part of the Children's Department of the Joint (Bethlem Royal and Maudsley) Hospitals. Our senior staff all have major commitments to these other areas of work, and attend their own outside meetings too. The Unit's Planning Meeting therefore acts also as a forum for noting, responding to and playing a part in 'outside' developments. Containing all this and more in a six-weekly meeting lasting an hour and a half is a challenge for chairman and members. Unlike our staff groups (Chapters 17 and 21) it is a decision-making meeting, and minutes are recorded.

These are just a few of the procedures we use, developed (and pruned) as the Unit has grown, and they are efficient and effective enough in aiding communication and recording information, including details of resources. Even the maintenance of the simple admission and discharge registers has prompted many prospective researchers to get a project off the ground before proceeding to more sophisticated methods.

I have welcomed my involvement in developing these approaches; what can be more demanding is my responsibility to help maintain them, especially as new staff in training come and go.

During the course of the average working day, if there is such a thing, the secretary doing this sort of work will be faced with a multitude of situations which require expertise and skills beyond the basic secretarial ones. She will need flexibility, tolerance and also a sense of humour.

A (nearly) typical day

9.00 am   Collect keys and mail from ward; distribute mail; open up cabinets.

9.15 am   Panic – keys to photocopying/coffee room won't work – ask round to see if other keys will work – call for carpenter. 3 telephone calls.

Consultant arrives for Ward Round; rest of staff collect messages and assemble for ward round.

Carpenter arrives – opens up room

9.30 am   Liaise with Nursing Officer over programme for Visitors Day. Start hospitality arrangements for Visitors Day – send out invitations to those attending, etc. 3 more calls for various people.

10.00 am   Mother of ex-inpatient telephones; wants help with other daughter, but not sure what help she wants. Spend 10 minutes listening – suggest she sees GP in first instance but will pass on message to Consultant and invite her to ring back after seeing GP. Get out notes of other daughter, type out message and leave for Consultant. More calls on internal and external lines. Coffee.

10.30 am   Sort out new referrals folder in preparation for Referrals Meeting. 3 more telephone calls – everyone in ward round, messages taken. (1 telephone call – Switchboard don't know where the person works; do we know?)
Social Worker wants Section papers. Ring through to Admin. to check on new procedure. Can't find patient notes relating to the section – ring round wards, check offices – not in ward round – notes eventually found. A patient strays in from another ward, lost. She, too, is found.

11.15 am   Break from Ward Round – staff in and out for messages, making coffee. Taking messages – giving out work, files, messages.

11.30 am   Routine typing of summaries; with various telephone calls.

12.30 pm   Ward Round finishes – Registrars leave management decisions to be typed.

1.00 pm   Lunch in Staff Dining Room. Consultant asks can we meet fairly quickly after lunch, and can the papers for the Section be brought to him.

2.00 pm   Meet with Consultant, go over his appointments; take any necessary work. Dictation over tricky staff problem. Interruption – Social Worker says mother won't sign her part of the Section papers. Brief discussion on how to go about this – back to dictation – take work back to own office; tactfully ease out two staff having a clinical discussion there.

2.45 pm   Psychologist says telephone not working – ring maintenance on another line. Nurses collecting for staff leaving present. A wants to speak to B. Where is he? Telephone calls; taking messages.
Cup of Tea.

3.30 pm   Urgent letter needs to go with Section papers – done direct onto typewriter – signed and sent off.

3.45 pm   Nurse comes and says change of plan re farewell drink next week – can we let staff know on the News-sheet.
Teacher comes in to ask if report re school placement been done by Registrar. Notes checked, not been done, message left for Registrar.

4.15 pm   Diary set up for next week.
Plants arrive from Gardens for Reception and Ward – distributed.

4.45 pm   Admin ring; have Section papers been done?
Various telephone calls.

5 pm   Finish, just.

★   ★   ★

All this is not everyone's cup of tea; temporary secretaries have been known to stay for only a few hours and then decide that they have had enough. On the other hand, some temporary secretaries have worked on the Unit and then stayed for a long time; staff have worked here for 25 years as well as for one day. As for me, my time here has been just about half way between the two extremes. Working as a secretary on the Adolescent Unit has its rewards, not least because of the recognition by my colleagues of the special role of the secretaries in a large and complex team.

The Adolescent Unit
Edited by Derek Steinberg
© 1986 John Wiley & Sons Ltd

14 The Chaplain

John Foskett

I am an anglican priest and hospital chaplain to the Bethlem Royal and Maudsley Hospitals. I read theology at Cambridge University, and have worked in parishes, youth organisations and therapeutic communities as well as in hospitals. My present work involves the training and supervision of students and colleagues on courses in pastoral care and counselling, in staff group work and mental health consultation. I have worked with the Richmond Fellowship, the Tavistock Clinic children's and adolescent's department and the Westminster Pastoral Foundation. I am interested in developing the chaplain's ministry to groups and institutions as well as to individuals, and believe that theology has much to contribute in this area. The major themes of Judeo-Christian tradition, for instance, sin, salvation, redemption, atonement, grace, law, works, faith, incarnation and transcendence, once liberated from their stereotyped ecclesiology, are powerful symbols for understanding the problems and possibilities facing society today. I am involved in contemporary movements which questions traditional assumptions about politics and power, and the traditional institutions of medicine, law and religion. I am married and have four adolescent children.

Recent books on adolescent psychiatry and psychology have had little if anything to say about religion's contribution to human growth and development. Although this might be expected, a sign of secularisation in society (Wilson, B. 1969), it is evidence of a significant change. In previous generations in western society, and still in some societies, the transition from child to adult was always accompanied by a religious ritual, such as barmitzvah or confirmation. Today only small minorities value these rites, and of those who do many believe that they are best undergone later, at the 'coming of age' of the adolescent. This is a reminder of how the step from child to adult has grown in the last hundred years, and may be stretched still further with greater unemployment. Today the change from dependance to independence is a lengthy procedure, and there are no accompanying sacraments to help acknowledge and contain its tensions and uncertainties.

These changes must in part account for the numbers of adolescents who find their way to psychiatric clinics and units. Is there anything which religion can offer to help what is no longer a single step but a considerable journey for adolescents? That is the question which this chapter seeks to address.

According to Levine (1979), 'Adolescents have two basic psychological needs, which when fulfilled enable them to cope better with those critical years and thereafter. These are, simply put, *a belief system* (his italics), something intense to believe in, and *a sense of belonging*, or community.' The following examples show something of the change mentioned above, and demonstrate how religion can help and hinder adolescents in meeting their basic needs to believe and to belong.

> 'Now his parents went to Jerusalem every year at the feast of the Passover. And when he was twelve years old, they went up according to custom; and when the feast was ended, as they were returning, the boy Jesus stayed behind in Jerusalem. His parents did not know it, but supposing him to be in the company they went a day's journey, and they sought him among their kinsfolk and acquaintances; and when they did not find him, they returned to Jerusalem, seeking him. After three days they found him in the temple, sitting among the teachers, listening to them and asking them questions; and all who heard him were amazed at his understanding and his answers. And when they saw him they were astonished; and his mother said to him, "Son, why have you treated us so? Behold, your father and I have been looking for you anxiously." And he said to them, "How is it that you sought me? Did you not know that I must be in my Father's house?" And they did not understand the saying which he spoke to them. And he went down with them and came to Nazareth, and was obedient to them; and his mother kept all these things in her heart.' *St Luke*

St Luke's story captures the flavour of adolescence, of worried parents and self absorbed and questioning youngsters. It also shows how the adolescent Jesus goes about resolving his emotional and spiritual needs. He already has freedom of movement within his extended family. What is more he is not afraid to search for belief and belonging in a place which includes both, and which belongs to his parents as much as to him. Although they do not understand his behaviour Mary is able to contain her fears, 'to keep (or treasure) all these things in her heart.' There is a temple, a faith, a community and so a structure within which growth and change can take place.

The second example is an account by a contemporary mother of her fourteen year old daughter's response to being asked to write about God, including how she would tell a young child about Him.

'For a start, I think it is all in the mind.' She went on to explain that she thinks God is your conscience: a voice inside telling you what sort of person you ought to be.

On the question of talking about God to a child, she revealed what I can only describe as a genuine anger. She says she doesn't know how you can talk about God to a child without causing it to misunderstand. 'How can a child not think God is an actual person in a place called Heaven, when everyone talks about him as 'Him'. Even in church, where you expect them to tell the truth. They pray to him as if he were a person, and even put him where you can see him in stained glass windows. . . . You don't know what to think. You feel you have been cheated with fairy stories, which the grown-ups still apparently believe and, at the same time, you feel guilty because you can't believe them yourself.'

She now finds herself at the point where she is beginning to understand that grown ups *don't* believe this, nor did they expect her to believe it in this literal way. It has all been a complete misunderstanding, hence her bitter cri-di-coeur. 'But just think of all those years when I *thought* I didn't believe in God!' (Robinson 1966).

The Psychiatric Unit and the Chaplain

Child and adult today encounter transition and change without the support of an all-embracing structure, temple, faith or community upon which to rely while beliefs are worked out and fellowship found. There are many reasons why adolescents and their parents consult psychiatric units and clinics, but it is my belief, based upon observation of one such unit and use of another, that a part of their quest is for something akin to the 'temple'. A place where the search for belief and belonging is acknowledged, questions attended to and anxiety contained.

The other chapters in this book have outlined the 'dimensions', 'rituals', and 'services' of this 'temple', and of how they are combined in order to create an atmosphere productive of health and wholeness. Medicine, the behavioural sciences, social and educational theories have all been harnessed to help in this enterprise. Somewhere a long the line religion and theology have been left behind, and with them a wealth of knowledge about 'temples' has been mislaid. For the unit or clinic which wants to reclaim some of those lost resources, the chaplain is a potential asset. In the rest of this chapter I will explore the problems and possibilities of utilising the chaplain's resources.

The National Health Service employs chaplains, Jewish, Roman Catholic, Free Church and Church of England, in all its hospitals. They are paid by the health service and licensed by their respective religious authorities. The majority are local clergy or rabbis, who give only a part of their time to chaplaincy work. Larger hospitals including many mental illness and handicap hospitals have full time C. of E. chaplains. Although chaplains are not usually appointed to psychiatric clinics, the clinics themselves are situated near to churches and synagogues, and many local clergy would recognise a pastoral responsibility to a clinic if their services were sought.

The first step for any unit, and I will use unit to mean clinic as well, interested in pursuing this would be to meet their hospital chaplains or local clergy, either by inviting them to the unit or sharing in a seminar on some mutually interesting subject. Some hospitals provide training in pastoral care for clergy, which can include their placement as student chaplains on hospital wards. This is often a good way to overcome the inevitable anxieties of staff and chaplains, and allows each to learn from the other. Psychiatric staff for example can fear that chaplains will be missionaries rather than pastors, and chaplains can be awed by the professionalism of everyone else. The training they will have already received can vary enormously. Some will have no specialist qualifications, while others will have training as pastoral counsellors, psychotherapists, psychologists and social workers. Obviously they should not be expected to work beyond the limits of their expertise, and it is always best if they can share in the in-service training and supervision of the unit itself.

The pastoral care and counselling movement (APCC) can provide helpful advice on these matters and on the role of the chaplain. The movement began in the context of psychiatric institutions in the USA before the second world war, and has developed rapidly in the United Kingdom in the last ten years. It aims to relate theology to the social sciences, and the theory of pastoral care with the practice of it, using methods of training and supervision similar to those of social work and therapy. In particular, it has helped to reinforce the distinctiveness of the pastor's role as one of 'presence', of 'being' rather than 'doing'. Within the health service this is a unique role, which other professions have in part, but which can become obscured by all the things which have to be done. Because they are not primarily concerned with either pathology or treatment, chaplains can symbolise a concern for health as much as sickness, and for people as much as for patients and staff, which will help reinforce the reality that health is more than an absence of illness (Wilson 1975).

Referrals and Other Work

Patients can refer themselves

Chaplains who are able to *be* in the above sense will soon be approached by patients, much in the way they are in the community. The following is a real example of the kind of conversation which might take place:

Patient: Are you the chaplain?
Chaplain: Yes, I am.
Patient: Can I talk to you?
Chaplain: Yes, you can. Where shall we go?
Patient: Oh, somewhere outside I think . . . You're a bit like my dad. He was big . . . I wanted to talk about him. I should have brought his picture.
Chaplain: You sound very fond of him.
Patient: Yes, I am. Do you believe in life after death?
Chaplain: Mm?
Patient: I think about it a lot. Sometimes I feel he's very close, like in the cemetery. There's not a proper stone, because he was cremated; and also in my mum's bedroom. But not here in the hospital.
Chaplain: Not even when you look at his photograph?
Patient: That's funny, yes perhaps a bit then.
Chaplain: Do you talk to him?
Patient: No, that would be silly, wouldn't it?

Chaplain: Would it? You sound as though you did talk to him a lot when he was alive.

Patient: Yes, I did. He really looked after me. My Mum was out a lot. He was funny and he made me feel safe. He worried a lot about his health. Then it all happened so suddenly. He was in hospital and then he was dead.

Chaplain: That must have been very hard for you.

Patient: I suppose it was, but I didn't take it in. I still don't think he is really dead and it's over six years ago, when I was ten. I think he's just on holiday and will come back any day. Do you think that's silly?

Chaplain: No, not silly; more confusing and strange for you.

Patient: I'm not sure you see. Sometimes I want to get in touch with him . . . what do you think about all that?

Chaplain: Do you mean through a spiritualist?

Patient: Yes, is that wrong?

Chaplain: You sound uncertain about it?

Patient: I think I want to hear his voice.

Chaplain: What do you want to hear him say?

Patient: I don't know. Something reassuring I suppose.

Chaplain: I think I can imagine that. You said that when he was alive he took care of you. I guess it's natural to want his help and comfort now.

Patient: I would like some guidance.

Chaplain: From people like me or spiritualists? Do you think we may be able to get closer to him or something?

Patient: I don't know really, it's something like that. It's weird like trying to hang on to him once he's gone. And you can't do that really, you've got to let them go.

Chaplain: Perhaps that's what feels so difficult. You need him and yet you've got to face that he's gone.

Patient: Mm (agreeing).

Chaplain: What do you think your dad would have to say to you at the moment, if he heard you talking like this?

Patient: I think he'd be sad about what had happened, what I've done. He'd be angry that I've got into such a mess. He'd say that if he'd been around it wouldn't have happened.

The patient went on to recall her feelings of guilt as well as sadness, and of how she needed to make up for missing the funeral, and then of getting into such a mess. She thought she had made a kind of confession, and wanted to go to a church and put it to God in her own words. Some months later the chaplain noticed the following entry above her name in the chapel intercession book.

'I would like to thank you, Lord, for giving me the strength to get better. Please, Lord, I would like you to forgive my sins, and make me a much wiser and better person.'

In this example the chaplain combines in one the roles of counsellor, pastor and priest. As counsellor his work is much the same as a therapist of any other discipline. As pastor he is the representative figure of religion's temple and faith. Elsewhere

I have explored the pastoral counsellor's contribution to the care of the mentally ill (Foskett 1984). As priest or religious specialist he can draw upon a great deal that we now know about the process of believing: of how people believe, as well as what they believe in. The patient in the conversation above was struggling with her beliefs; some were still quite childlike and others were beginning to take account of more mature ideas.

Goldman (1964) has made a study of the religious thinking of childhood and adolescence along lines similar to those of Piaget. The religious thinking of children up to the age of seven is intuitive and lacks reasoning and consistency. A young child when asked why Moses was afraid of God at the burning bush said 'God had a funny face and a horrid voice'. From eight to twelve a child's thinking becomes more concrete and operational; reason, logic and consistency are more in evidence. For a child of this age, 'Moses is frightened because he thinks God will chase him off the holy ground, because he has not taken his shoes off.' From thirteen onwards abstract religious though begins to develop. Adolescents can think hypothetically and deductively, and can reason symbolically as well as literally; so that 'Moses is frightened because God is awesome and almighty, and makes him feel like a worm.' Despite the work of Goldman and others (Lee 1965; Fowler 1981) many adolescents will have had little if any help with the development of their religious thinking. The young people who consult a psychiatric unit will have had many buffets to their belief systems, and more than perhaps anything else will need to reclaim and rediscover their capacity for faith. This is an area where chaplains can usefully co-operate with others, teachers and psychotherapists in particular, to identify where a young patient's beliefs have suffered the most, and how best to aid recovery. Patients of this age can so easily cling to false, illusory and simplistic beliefs. Some psychoses and most neuroses have this quality to them, as does attachment to extreme and often persecutory religious groups.

Staff can refer patients

This is especially likely when a patient is preoccupied with religious or moral questions, and like Jesus in the temple needs to find today's equivalent of a scribe or Pharisee. It is important that staff have the patient's permission before they refer him to the chaplain. Alternatively they can consult the chaplain themselves in order to clarify the best way to proceed. For instance an agnostic teacher was very perplexed by a patient's attempts to get her to discuss heaven and hell; after consulting the chaplain she felt more able to help her pupil explore these issues for herself.

Life events and crises

The traumata of major life events, especially involving the death of a patient, one of their relatives or a member of staff, need adequate recognition. Meetings can be arranged to help staff and patients with their grief, and the chaplain's presence, more than what he says or does, can be very important. He can facilitate mourning by helping staff use an appropriate formal or informal ritual, such as a memorial or thanksgiving service. Services of this kind are best arranged to allow for the different beliefs, assumptions and needs of all who are likely to attend. For instance, a memorial service for an agnostic member of staff, whose family were Jewish, and who had many practising Christian friends, included contributions from all these points of view. In the same way, the chaplain can help with the celebration of events like births and marriages. The more the chaplain can involve others in the planning of their rituals the more it will meet their needs, and help them to retain contact with the wider world at a time when circumstances may make them feel isolated and alone.

The care of staff

Hospital chaplains are now appointed to minister to staff as much as to patients, but at first staff may be cautious about approaching the chaplain in a context where they are supposed to be the helpers. Committed believers are likely to turn to their own minister for help, but some at least may look to the chaplain and fellow believers for support with the tensions of faith and action in their work. Staff religious fellowships as well as individual meetings with the chaplain are useful for this.

For all staff, irrespective of their beliefs, chaplains are possible confidants. Their neutral position within the institution and its hierarchies means they can be used as counsellors for a whole range of issues to do with work and life as well as with religion.

Ethical matters

The practitioners of psychiatry and psychology are committed, like other scientists, to assessing the value and effectiveness of their work. Research as well as treatment and training raises ethical issues. The chaplain as 'outsider' to a unit can observe the assumptions and methods of the behavioural scientists with a layman's eye; as 'insider' he is familiar enough with disciplines to provide an informed critique of their work. It is likely that the health service will be required to become more answerable to society for what it does, and the need for some ethical forum will grow. The chaplain is an obvious focus for this work.

Moral and religious education

Patients and staff may wish to foster some exploration of the major issues of worth, value and morals, for example in the school. In the community at large churches and youth groups provide opportunities for young people to share and discuss these things, and the chaplain can be enlisted to help plan and organise similar meetings.

The Chaplain as a source of referral

As representatives of their religion or denomination, chaplains are in contact with an extensive social network in the community. With social workers and community nurses they can help to retain or make contacts between the institution and the outside world, including people who may want help.

Conclusions

Enough has been said to illustrate the ways in which chaplains can make a useful and effective contribution to the work of an adolescent unit. Nevertheless, there may continue to be important questions and doubts in the minds of both staff and chaplains; patients usually work these out for themselves. The lack of a defined role can create anxiety, especially in a tense and confusing context. Like all anxiety it is a mixed blessing. Concern and curiosity about the chaplain's motives can help bring into sharper relief the motives of all who work on a unit. The hidden beliefs and assumptions which all helpers bring to their work can be usefully teased out into the open, and the unit begin to assess the helpful and harmful aspects of its belief systems. Teachers can question the value of their teaching, nurses of nursing and psychotherapists of their therapy. The effect of a chaplain's beliefs and motives should be no more and no less open to scrutiny than those of anyone else; but it may easier to start with the chaplains (Jung 1933). As was said earlier there is more to believing than the objects of belief. The chaplain's experience in this area can help a unit recognise the hidden faith or faiths upon which its work is founded. Halmos (1965) in his study of the helping professions included psychiatrists, psychologists and social workers within his general term 'counsellor', and wrote of them:

> 'By perservering in his efforts to help, the counsellor seems to make a point, take a stand, and declare for hope. At a time when, according to all common sense standards the client appears incorrigibly useless the counsellor is, in fact, saying 'you are worthwhile', and 'I am not put off by your illness.' This moral stance of not admitting defeat is possible only for those who have a faith or a kind of stubborn confidence in the rightness of what they are doing. . . . On the whole the counsellors are frankly and humbly agnostic, and for this reason their much restrained piety is plausible and acceptable in the sceptical age in which they have to work. Yet they use a language of reverence, and even a theological language and imagery, as if they could not do their job effectively without their evocative power.'

A mature or maturing faith is as important to an adolescent as is emotional and intellectual maturity. Many of those who seek the help of a psychiatric unit will have little or no faith left, and will test the faith of their helpers to the utmost. The chaplain can help a unit own and value the beliefs that its work has honed and refined, especially at those times when it feels most faithless and hopeless. Near the end of his life Maslow (1979) put it like this:

'I'd always assumed . . . that if you cleared away the rubbish and the neurosis and the garbage and so on, then the person would blossom out, that he'd find his own way. I find especially with the young people that it just ain't so sometimes. That is, it's possible to be loved and respected, etc. and even so to feel cynical and materialistic and to feel there is nothing worth working for . . . Especially in the younger rather than the older people you can see this. It's sort of a loss of nerve, and I think we're at this point where the traditional culture has broken down altogether, and for many people they just feel, "My God, there is nothing".'

Much of the work and activity of an adolescent unit can be a defence against facing that anxiety. Patients will bring this despair, put it down at the feet of the staff and watch carefully what is done with it. Chaplains can be equally threatened and reply defensively, 'There's not nothing, there's God.' But equally they can draw upon their theological traditions, and meet these questions not with easy answers or distracting activity, but with patience and acceptance. In being present with the sick and the troubled and with those who care for them, the chaplain confesses to the truth that faith given a chance, can grow out of doubt and despair, and that such a faith really does belong to and enliven those who come to believe in it.

References and Further Reading

APCC (1973) *The Constitutional Papers of the Association for Pastoral Care and Counselling.* These and other details can be obtained from the British Association for Counselling, 37a Sheep Street, Rugby, Warwickshire

Foskett J H (1984) *Meaning in Madness,* Pastoral Counselling and Psychiatry SPCK London.

Fowler J (1981) *The Stages of Faith.* New York: Harper & Row

Goldman R (1964) *Religious Thinking from Childhood to Adolescence.* London: Routledge & Kegan Paul

Goldman R (1965) *Readiness for Religion.* London: Routledge & Kegan Paul

Halmos P (1965) *The Faith of the Counsellors.* London: Constable

Jung C G (1933) *Modern Man in Search of a Soul.* London: Routledge & Kegan Paul

Jung C G (1977) *Memories, Dreams and Reflections.* London: Collins

Jung C G (1964) *Man and his Symbols.* London: Aldus Books

Lee R S (1965) *Your Growing Child and Religion.* Harmondsworth: Penguin Books

Levine S (1979) Adolescents believing and belonging. In S C Feinstein & P L Giovacchini (eds) *Adolescent Psychiatry, Vol 7.* University of Chicago Press

Luke St *Gospel According to,* 2.41-51, Revised Standard Version

Maslow A (1979) A quotation from an interview with William Frick. In *Theology,* 82(685), 18-19.

Other Faiths SPCK (1983) *Our Ministry and Other Faiths.* London: Church House

Robinson R (1966) *Seventeen Come Sunday.* London: SCM Press

Wilson B (1969) *Religion in a Secular Society.* Harmondsworth: Penguin

Wilson M (1975) *Health is for People.* London: Darton, Longman & Todd

15 Research and the Psychiatric Professions

Eric Taylor

I took a psychology degree in 1965 and medical degree in 1968. After that I did a number of house jobs at the Middlesex, Central Middlesex and other London hospitals in psychiatry, neurology, and various medical specialties. I then spent 1971/72 as a research and clinical fellow at Harvard University and Massachusetts General Hospital in Boston. A strong interest in the neurophysiological basis of behaviour took me into research with hyperactive children, and this has remained my main research activity. In 1973 I came to the Maudsley for training in psychiatry and child psychiatry and in 1978 I began a career post as Senior Lecturer at the Institute of Psychiatry. This involves clinical child psychiatry and the teaching of child psychiatry and child development to several disciplines; but it also allows me to spend time in research. I am engaged in several different kinds of study - clinical, epidemiological and cross-cultural - to try to understand the nature of the problems of childhood hyperactivity and attention deficit. I also combine a research and a clinical interest in the problems of adolescents who attempt suicide.

———◆———

'Research' can mean many things. At one extreme of the spectrum is the small number of teams of full-time researchers pursuing a major programme of scientific investigation and addressing themselves primarily to the international scientific community. At the other end is the part-time (perhaps even spare-time) investigation by an unaided health worker – making, perhaps, an evaluation of his own practice, or checking on a clinical hunch. Both kinds of work, and many intermediate forms, are essential. In a healthy professional community there will be a continuum of scale of enterprises.

Sometimes 'research' is spoken of by clinicians as though it were quite apart from or even opposed to the world in which patients seek help from therapists. In fact, research in the sense of systematic enquiry is a necessary part of clinical practice. The habit of mind that critically tests ideas against evidence is as necessary in the consulting room as in the laboratory. Unfortunately, however, professional researchers have often become somewhat separated from the clinical professions. This chapter will try to describe something of the background to research work and its complex relationship with the practice of psychiatry.

147

Characteristics of Scientific Work

The volume and prestige of 'big science' have expanded enormously through the course of the century. Adolescent psychiatry has so far been less influenced by it than almost any other branch of medicine. Even now, however, no practitioner can afford to ignore the methods and findings of researchers. The future is very likely to bring more, and more clinically relevant, investigations.

Several of the characteristics of scientists follow from the expansion of science. Specialisation, for example, becomes a necessity. This can be seen simply as a consequence of the mass of information and techniques that has to be mastered. One index of this is the number of scientific papers published in a given field. Generally speaking, the number rises exponentially as years go by; not only does it increase, but the *rate* of increase also rises. By contrast, the number of scientists working in a given field has tended to rise much more slowly and steadily; and cutbacks in recent years have often halted the growth. Yet papers do *not* get simpler, and people do not get cleverer. The quantity of information with which each scientist must cope is therefore itself increasing. One way of managing this is for researchers to confine themselves to ever more restricted subject areas.

If specialisation went unchecked, it could be a disastrous trend. Advances in knowledge often come when ideas from superficially different areas are brought together. If investigations were to become steadily more restricted in scope, then one would have to expect them to grow more and more arid. One of the ways in which this trend is checked is through multidisciplinary collaboration. Teams of investigators with different kinds of expertise join to work on a common problem. This in itself can create difficulties. For one thing, it is expensive; for another, who gets the credit? Nevertheless, the difficulties have to be overcome. The romantic idea of a single outstanding individual 'voyaging through strange seas of thought, alone' bears little relationship to today's teamwork and research industries.

Other characteristics of scientific investigation follow directly from the nature of the activity. Evidently, it is trying to pose and answer unsolved questions; and the answers may well not be in keeping with conventional wisdom. If the accepted tenets of the clinical professions were always true, then there would be little need for research. Accordingly, recruits need to be independently-minded, self-critical, and prepared, if necessary, to follow unpopular lines. A perfectly organised profession would therefore provide for considerable independence in its members.

The need to understand clinical problems in new ways also means that researchers' work has to be replicable. The goal is to develop public knowledge that did not exist before. The yardstick by which one judges whether public knowledge has been achieved is whether other people can find the same result. I do not mean to claim that the human sciences can or should achieve a complete and wholly public account of the nature of people's problems. This is probably an impossible goal (Ziman 1978). Nevertheless, the strong practical need to have some shared knowledge means that researchers have to put great effort into achieving reliable measures. The only way to ensure that somebody else will get the same results with the same method is to make the method as faithful as possible a reflection of the phenomena. Research measures, therefore, must often be much more time-consuming than clinical evaluations. It is harder to convince other people than oneself. By the same token, research measures are often less rich and extensive than clinical assessments, at least in the early stages of development. The attainment of reliability can be so very time-consuming that the focus of enquiry must be limited.

The data gathering that researchers do is consequently painstaking, craftsmanlike and patient. Like craftsmen, they need to take pride in the successful and consistent performance of unglamorous work. The time required for it is great, and this is one of the major obstacles in the way of clinical workers who want to share in research activity.

The working relationships between researchers are also in part a consequence of the historical forces mentioned above and the economic constraints considered below. Because researchers are generally independent and autonomous people, and because they need to collaborate with others, they often relate in informal groups with little attention to the disciplines to which individuals belong. Because basic and clinical scientists work together yet clinicians are paid more, there is a real potential for friction.

Researchers are usually rather competitive. Success is often measured largely by grants won and papers published. Resources are harshly limited, so that survival requires a continuing ability to win the competitions that determine the allocation of money. The judges for the race are essentially other scientists: those who sit on funding bodies or review for them, and the editors and referees of scientific journals. It should be no surprise that disputes and tensions can arise about the credit for some pieces of work.

Finally, scientific work bearing on the psychiatry of childhood and adolescence has an important extra characteristic. It is scanty. The subject is beginning. Researchers are few.

Organisation and Funding of Research

Because major projects require specialist teams, they are expensive; and the management and funding of research therefore become crucial. Nobody knows exactly how it should be organised. Many of the most productive laboratories in other subjects have managed to combine a clear common purpose with considerable autonomy for individual workers. A balance has to be kept, if we are to avoid the hazards on the one hand of a fragmented set of secure individuals whose work is self-indulgent or does not communicate with others; and on the other hand of a research proletariat who labour on specific projects without the chance to use their own creativity.

This need for balance between generalised research and specific investigations has led to most governmental support being channelled through a binary system (Himsworth 1970). The universities provide a system of established, long-term teaching posts, equipment and resources for investigations, and students learning the trade. The research councils provide funds for specific projects seeking to answer a limited question, for whole units exploring a specified field of enquiry, and for the support and training of individal researchers. The two systems were generally seen as working tolerably well together; but university cuts in recent years have distorted the balance and there may be a heavy price to pay.

The National Health Service itself spends relatively little money on research, at least by comparison with other science-based industries. Historically, this resulted from the wish to have an independent scheme of funding through research councils lest the innovative value of research should be compromised by the administrative policies of Ministers eager that research findings should not upset their plans (HMSO 1919). Nevertheless, the Department of Health and Social Services commissions some research, especially about the operation of the Health Services rather than the nature of disorders. Further, all regional health authorities have a budget for research, and one purpose of this is precisely to encourage local initiatives and small-scale enquiries.

Commercial bodies, such as drug firms, also commission research but so far this has contributed only little to child and adolescent psychiatry in the UK. Independent charitable foundations (such as the Mental Health Fund, Wellcome Trust and Ciba Foundation) have an importance out of proportion to their size. They have much less money to spend than, say, their American counterparts, but they are able to be flexible and innovative in their policies, and perhaps even able to take more risks than governmentally-funded agencies.

The universities therefore have a particularly important role in developing psychiatric research. They expanded in the 1960s and now have to face serious cutbacks. The position of young researchers is therefore precarious. In the absence of career posts their incomes usually have to come from short-term grants for specific projects. There is a real danger that many will leave academic work, and that those who remain will be prevented from the general development of their subject by the need to devote themselves to immediate project work. The academic community is therefore ageing.

Training of Researchers

After taking their degree, people who plan a pure research career spend several years (usually three to five) in postgraduate training. This leads to a PhD degree, and most of it is spent in carrying out a research project under supervision. Their research immediately thereafter will probably be in postdoctoral fellowships or in working as research assistants; their goal is usually a permanent post in a university department or a research unit.

In a sense, this is a straightforward and well-mapped path. However, many people come to research from different routes, and it is highly desirable that they should be able to do so, bringing with them a variety of approaches and kinds of expertise. Furthermore, many who are clinicians by vocation can and should pursue systematic investigations, and therefore should have access to research training. In some disciplines, particularly clinical psychology and psychiatry, the successful completion of a small project is a key part of the clinical training and is pursued part-time. This gives at least an appreciation of the approach, and is a good basis for a more systematic training. The best way of taking this further is through a period of full-time supervised research on a training fellowship, or as a research assistant. There has been recent criticism of this kind of training (Culliton 1984). A year or two may be simply not long enough to train as an independent investigator. Physicians who have taken this pathway through the (American) National Institutes of Health are not likely to obtain further research grants on graduating. While this may be a caution, I do not think that it applies to a subject that is as underdeveloped, in research terms, as psychiatry. There is a great deal of basic work to be done in describing the patterns of disorder and charting their course. Great sophistication is not yet necessary for advancing knowledge, and the amateur still has a crucial part to play.

Interactions Between Clinic and Academy

When clinicians and researchers are out of touch with each other unhelpful attitudes and stereotypes can grow, unchecked by reality. People working wholly for the Health Service can come to imagine that their researching colleagues are dilettanti, or magicians, or heartlessly self-seeking, or dangerous rivals. Academics can suppose that the clinical professions are complacent, with vested interests in maintaining the status quo.

Shaffer (1976) made a survey of all the research going on at that time in the UK in the fields of child and adolescent psychiatry. He concluded that excellent work was being carried out, but that there was a serious lack of a research base. Developmental psychology was proceeding in isolation from psychiatry, and lacking in guidance or stimulation from it. Clinical research was skewed towards the study of mild or uncommon conditions. This bias might have been a result of the powerful influence of paediatrics, and a diversion of attention from the common, and often serious, emotional disorders and disorders of conduct which make up most of the morbidity in the community. Ten years later, the comment would require some modification. Links are steadily increasing. Nevertheless, full collaboration is still a rare thing.

One obvious link is that research provides information that clinicians need, but this should not be overstated. Scientific findings do not tell a psychiatrist exactly how he should treat a case. Every individual is different, and art as well as science is required to make one's knowledge about groups of people relevant to a single case. Even when clear lessons can be drawn from reliable findings, clinicians do not necessarily change their practice to fit. To alter the treatment of one condition may entail difficult changes in the social structure of clinics. Suppose, for instance, that individual counselling were repeatedly shown to be harmful in the long term for antisocial teenagers. This is a hypothetical example, which could be true under some circumstances (McCord 1978). Clinicians who use the treatment would then be faced by a suggestion that their practice should alter radically. Most would look very critically indeed at how far the results could be generalised to their own clientele and their own kind of therapy. Nevertheless, and in spite of the difficulties in interpretation, the findings of research constitute the maps to which clinicians refer in their exploration of the unknown territory of a new case.

This leads to another kind of link between clinical and research workers. Clinical workers are an important part of the audience for research, and their expectations will guide the kind of investigations that are done. At one level this is obvious: questions from the clinic need research answers. Does, for example, family therapy add anything to behaviour treatment in helping children with school refusal? The practical importance of the question makes it likely that a formal trial of treatments would have some priority in the allocation of research funds. More subtly, the precise form of the question will be governed by current clinical wisdom. If, for example, the general consensus was that family therapy was a standard treatment and the best available, then the question might well need to be changed to 'Does behavioural treatment add anything to family therapy?' If the two treatments are conceived of as rivals, the question might be 'Is family therapy better than behavioural treatment?'

At another level, even the technical details of the research will be influenced by what the audience expects. In our imaginary example of a direct comparison of behaviour therapy and family therapy, a decision would have to be taken about how children are allocated to one treatment or another. One way of doing it would be to make it entirely random. Another way would be to 'stratify', ie. to ensure that the two groups are well matched and that no treatment is favoured unfairly by being given to a better-prognosis group. Statisticians and experimentalists disagree among themselves about which strategy is better. The answer seems to be that the better strategy is that which will be more persuasive to its target audience (Brown 1980). Science is a social activity. The sophistication of its consumers will in part determine what is done.

Another kind of relationship arises when a clinician seeks to learn from a researcher. He might ask for supervision on a research project or for consultation in the design of a study. If this is to be useful, then each side needs a good working understanding of the other. Problems sometimes arise when expectations are unrealistically high. A clinician may, for instance, hope that there will be ready technical answers when in fact the questions are difficult ones of substance that need to be tackled conceptually. The following sketch is imaginary, but the misunderstanding is real and common.

Clinician **(C)**   The team would be very grateful if you would help us with the details of starting a study about how best to treat our school refusers.

Researcher **(R)**   I'll be glad to try. What study were you planning to do?

C   Well, that was what I was asking really. Most of us are working in family-orientated ways but we are not clear about whether it is making any real difference. What outcome measures are there for us to use?

R   Before talking about measures I'd need to be clearer about what you intend to change. Do you plan to have a group receiving no treatment?

C   No, that doesn't seem ethical.

R   Then you won't really be able to know whether your treatment is making any difference beyond doing nothing. Look, I can't help you much until you know what issue you want to examine. I think it would be better if you were to sit down and write out an outline of what you want to do.

C   I was hoping that you'd be doing that.

Both sides in the dialogue have under-rated the difficulty and key importance of the very first step in a scientific investigation: the formulating of a useful and answerable question. This usually involves a whole process of refining the issue, rethinking it, and making it both more precise and more restricted. It may well be more sensible to ask an experienced researcher to join in the early discussions that formulate a problem, than to seek only technical help.

This may lead on to the closest relationship between academic workers and the clinical professions, that of full collaboration on projects. The clearest instances of the benefits and problems in such an association comes from conducting clinical trials. This brings a real clash between the needs and philosophies of the two disciplines. On the one side is the research requirement that the treatment to be given is as precisely specified as possible and that individual subjects are treated alike except for the experimental intervention to be assessed. On the other side is the determination of clinicians that their patients will be treated in the best possible way for them, individually tailored to their circumstances.

The dilemma is as much practical as ethical. The ethics seem to depend upon how clearly clinicians know that their treatments work. If they simply do not know whether a particular intervention is helpful, then the most ethical way of giving it is in the manner that allows knowledge to develop most securely. Uncontrolled experiments are therefore worse than formal trials. When, by contrast, there is a firm clinical conviction that a treatment is effective then there are real ethical problems in withholding it from people who need help. Even when the ethical decision is made and a trial is started, there may still be an emotional problem for therapists if they dislike one of the treatments to which their clients may be committed.

Consider again the fictitious example of a randomised trial of family therapy against behaviour modification in the treatment of school refusal. Perhaps it has been agreed that the therapists will determine whether potential subjects are in fact suitable and, if so, allocate them to the next treatment on a randomised list. The therapists would then be under strong internal pressure to fiddle the procedure so that their client gets the treatment that they feel he needs most. This might or might not be in the client's best interest, but it would certainly distort the ability of the trial to give a clear and replicable answer.

Collaborating in a trial therefore requires much flexibility from clinicians. They have to accept that, for its duration, they lose some of their freedom of manoeuvre. The possible reward is that, after the trial, they will have a far clearer understanding of what they do, and a way of communicating precisely with other therapists. It is urgent that this form of collaboration should develop.

How Will Research Help?

Nobody knows how systematic investigations will change the practice of child and adolescent psychiatry. If it were known, they would not need to be done. It is all the harder to guess the future when research is only at the beginning of exploring the subject.

Nevertheless, the experience of other disciplines suggests a few clear lessons. Exposure to systematic research will help clinicians in their acquisition of the skills of critical testing of ideas, and towards scepticism and tolerance in their theoretical frameworks. This is wholly compatible with the need to make clear decisions, even in relative ignorance. Indeed, the charting of what is known and unknown should be an asset. Sceptics can also be optimists about the value of their treatments. Finally, research is likely to accelerate the rate of change. This will certainly put new strains upon clinical workers; it will also save their disciplines from atrophy.

References and Further Reading

Brown B W B Jr (1980) Statistical Controversies in the Design of Clinical Trials - Some Personal Views. *Controlled Clinical Trials*, **1**, 13-27

Culliton B (1984) NIH starts review of training programs. *Science*, **223**, 194-196

His Majesty's Stationery Office (1919) *Memorandum on the Ministry of Health Bill, 1919, as to the Work of the Medical Research Committee.* Cmd 69. London: HMSO

Himsworth H (1970) *The Development and Organisation of Scientific Knowledge.* London: Heinemann

McCord J (1978) A thirty-year follow-up of treatment effects. *American Psychologist*, **33**, 284-289

Shaffer D (1976) *Child Behaviour Research: A Survey of British Research into Child Psychiatric Disorder and Normal Social Development: 1975/1976.* London: Medical Research Council

Ziman J (1978) *Reliable Knowledge: An Exploration of the Grounds for Belief in Science.* Cambridge: Cambridge University Press

16 Education for nurses: Support, Supervision, Training

Teresa Wilkinson

I began nurse training in August 1970 on a course leading to State Registration and the London University Diploma in Nursing. By the time I qualified as a general nurse I was interested in psychiatric nursing. My interest had been fostered through a psychiatric placement in a large institution, which caused me some distress, and through caring for patients admitted to a medical ward after attempting suicide or taking an accidental overdose. In both situations I felt inadequate in both skill and knowledge. My decision to train in psychiatric nursing was also political. I believed that all nurses should be doubly-trained to look after whole people so I put my beliefs to the test. I was accepted on a training scheme and resigned; then there was a mix up involving a six-month wait to start training, but I was offered staffing experience on the child psychiatric ward as a stop-gap. Not liking to withdraw my notice I accepted this offer with the proviso that if after a month I hated the children I would be moved! That was in January 1974 and it would seem that I didn't hate the children – I found them objectionable, loveable, tiring, aggressive pests, but I didn't hate 'it'. I left the children's ward to train as a Registered Mental nurse but had no doubt that I would go back to working with children. On completion of the course I obtained promotion to the post ward sister, child psychiatry, at the Maudsley. I have been associated with young people since that time – August 1975.

I first became interested in teaching nurses whilst working as a ward sister. That job is one of the most difficult within the nursing structure. It is a combination of direct patient care, ward management, supervision of juniors and the liaison between the ward nursing management and non-nurse team members. I noticed similarities between nursing interventions and teaching or supervision methods. The next profound thought was that I could influence the care of more young people by training others rather than by my own practice alone. My next and current job was organising the post-basic training course in Child and Adolescent Psychiatric Nursing. This was a new post and I enjoyed the challenge of setting up something new and trying out some of my ideas.

———◆———

To explore the support, supervision and training of nurses working with adolescents is the aim of this chapter, but I would first like to put it into the context of my job, tasks and belief system. The job involves organising the curriculum for a one year course for six trainees who are registered nurses with varying degrees of experience in the speciality. As well as curriculum planning I teach on the study days and supervise and teach in the clinical area. Selection and assessment of course members are partly my responsibility. Running a specialist course within a clinical area involves considerable liaison with the clinical team, which is multidisciplinary. Part of the task of working within a unit involves providing a service for the unit and not just taking from it for course members needs. To this end I participate in some staff groups, supervise specific clinical tasks and practice as a nurse in a small way.

I believe that to nurse young people formal training with children and adolescents is essential. It is important to put the behaviour of adolescents in the developmental context of where they have come from and where they are going. All trained psychiatric nurses have experience with adults but their experience with children and adolescents is very limited, and few have both. Participation in a formal course focuses both experience and theory to provide the practitioner with sound, holistic learning; one problem of personal study when working full time is that people are frequently too tired to read, and only rarely plan what they read and learn in a satisfactory and systematic way.

The aim of the course I organise is that its members will use the space for themselves in a way that provides them with not only knowledge and skills but the skill of organising their own learning to enable it to continue when the course finishes.

To achieve this I work within a framework of behavioural and cognitive objectives, some determined by myself as fitting the curriculum others defined personally by course members. Using objectives in this way allows the level of achievement to be tailored to the individual who devises ways of achieving learning and then identifies future learning objectives. Educationally, the principles of Gagne (1970), Bruner (1972) and Carl Rogers (1967) have influenced my practice. Learning is a multifaceted process; the individual uses many stimuli to organise his thinking, feelings and behaviour. Abercrombie (1970) described that process as being analagous to filling bottles: no bottle is empty, the bottles differ in size and the current contents will react to what is added. Learning is, therefore, an active process for the learner.

Structuring learning for nurses should make the learning quicker, more reliable, and more useful. The strategies used must reflect the learning process; for me this means that they should:

1 Involve the learner actively.
2 Have clear targets for the learners to aim for.
3 Involve cognition, behaviour and feelings.
4 Provide only as much as the learners need to stimulate their assimilation of the new whole.
5 Involve taking risks; it is impossible to predict the exact extent of learning.
6 Involve sharing with peers so that the process is 'live' and broad-based.

It also means for me that teachers should facilitate learning rather than give their own learning as a package to be accepted as a finite whole. Explaining learning can become long-winded and didactic, too. To combat this I will use a schematic diagram of learning cues from which, you, the reader can arrive at your own learning set which I hope will concur at some level with my own.

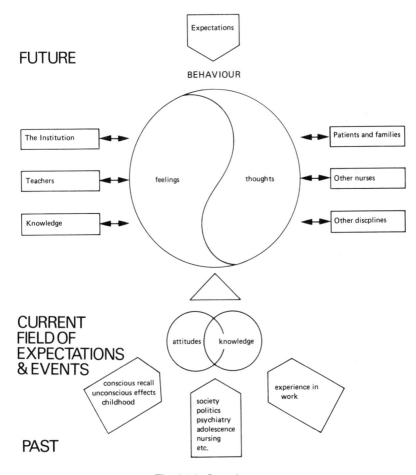

Fig. 16.1 Learning set

The role of the teacher is to explore with the learner the system outlined in the diagram. The explanation can be preplanned in a curriculum or instigated by the learners' immediate needs. By using a teacher the learner may avoid unnecessarily trailing around the system leading to anxiety and feeling deskilled and lost. My aim is to cover some areas involved in this explanation based principally on my own experiences. To do this I have divided the discussion into three broad categories:

Aspects of learning theory
Common problems
Strategies to assist learning

Aspects of Learning Theory

That no one can learn for someone else and that there are no short cuts to learning must be among the most hacknied truisms. The truth of this needs emphasising once again especially for nurses commencing post-basic courses, and perhaps for all professionals. The first feeling is that they know nothing; this, combined with the desire to help patients, quickly leads to a quest for answers. Previous work within a medical model often confirms a view that there is a 'right answer', and possibly a conspiracy to conceal it from them!

From the outset, learners need to accept certain principles, be motivated to learn, and recognise that there is not necessarily only one right answer to patients' problems. This is clearly demonstrated in the adolescent field where each discipline works within its own conceptual framework; often a variety of models are used within one discipline. The definition of problems depends on the conceptual framework used, which then dictates the type of treatment plan. In some teams an eclectic approach to definition and treatment is used, which means that models are used which seem to fit the presenting pattern. An early difficulty experienced by many professionals is in trying to fit an appealing model to problems not defined within the corresponding conceptual framework. Currently, family therapy is a popular model, and paradox an appealing intervention, but they are not universally applicable, an idea some new converts fail to appreciate. The idea of universality is not so prevalent with such established therapies as systematic desensitisation where experience and research have led to firm criteria for its use.

Choosing interventions which are suitable for the client and appropriate for the treatment is an exercise in problem solving, which is a cognitive skill. As a cognitive skill is learnt through practice, learners need to practise it and receive feedback which will refine their level of skill. Short cuts such as always asking more experienced colleagues works against the novice ever developing sound problem-solving skills. It is also worth remembering that the patient's failure to change is not always a consequence of faulty problem solving. It may be that the patient is resistant to change or that the prognosis is poor for some other reason.

A further principle can be described as exploring the raw material in the learning process. The learners are this raw material, and learning is influenced by their personality, past experience, cognitive ability, expectations and motivation. If one were filling up empty bottles responsibility for success would belong to the pourer. In a participant process, however, most of the responsibility falls to the learners, and they must be prepared to examine their approach to learning and therapeutic interventions. If the learners are unwilling to examine themselves, their failures (and successes) will be attributed to others. This projection removes the possibility of self-directed change and leaves the learner feeling impatient and frequently angry. Learners should work with the dilemma that learning imposes: that to accept personal responsibility involves risking painful as well as pleasureable experiences. The alternative, attributing responsibility to others can seem attractive but involves loss of autonomy and results in impotence and frustration.

For the psychiatric nurse (as for any other type of therapist) self-examination poses quite specific risks for the individual. I believe that some of these can be predicted, and it is the responsibility of the teacher to offer them to the learner to consider. By doing this the learners can make a decision about their preparedness to embark on learning. Withdrawal at this time is a positive comment on the learner's capacity for self-examination and should not be seen as failure. Agreement to enter a contract for learning, however, does not mean that all will be plain sailing; at many points the learner will be tempted to backtrack, alter the contract or withdraw. Risks that can be predicted include discovering (a) that we are not all capable of being the perfect therapist; (b) that our personalities can help or hinder learning and therapy; (c) that we all have different capacities to change as a result of learning; and (d) that our view of ourselves may be at variance with the view of others. Strategies to work with these risks include group discussion, role-playing predicted risk areas and individual counselling. A problem I have identified follows from the fact that nurses on post-basic courses are a self-selected group whose motivation to complete the course is high; the source of the motivation can vary from a desire to learn for oneself to being instructed to complete the course as a way of keeping a job or gaining promotion. The latter creates an anxiety and defensiveness which hinders learning.

Nurses not on courses have different problems. Primarily they have entered a contract to work in a certain place for a given period and there is no formal expectation from them to enter into structured learning. This makes it difficult to join with them in a process of discovery which will be uncomfortable at the very least. Often these nurses select only the more comfortable or personally interesting options and this does not give them a breadth of skill and empathy with the subjects of their interventions, who are expected to feel some discomfort as they change and become 'healthy'. Another problem for nurses contracted as workers is that even if they are prepared to enter a learning contract there is often little space in a programme designed primarily for direct patient care. Commonly there is a sense of guilt about taking time away from the adolescents to look after themselves. It is helpful if they can believe that productive time for self can dramatically increase the value of time spent with the adolescents. I would guess that nurses who spend all their time 'working' soon cease to be effective. When work involves using oneself as the therapeutic tool it must involve caring for and improving the tool.

Common Problems

In this section I will describe some of the dilemmas which have been presented to me by my course members and which I have observed in staff groups or experienced myself. I hope that my understanding of the problems will assist their resolution. I believe this occurs when the nurse understands the nature of an experience and uses that understanding to locate precisely where change is needed, rather than accepting responsibility for curing or changing everything.

Limit setting

Put crudely this is the ability to say 'no' to an adolescent's demands or behaviour. The dilemma frequently voiced is how does the nurse know when it is the right time to draw a line, what is fair and for the ultimate good of the young person? Occasionally these straightforward questions are about central problems around which learning takes place. More frequently, these questions are not the real issues. Often the nurse is caught between adhering to intellectual beliefs or following gut reactions which are a mixture of counter-transference and personal unconscious mechanisms.

Intellectual beliefs can be professionally based on nursing practice and developmental theory, or political and social. The latter may involve attitudes to democracy and individual freedom which run counter to the practice of limiting the adolescent's autonomy. Unconscious mechanisms can relate to past authority figures, the individual's own upbringing and current relationships. The countertransference is concerned with what the nurse accepts of the adolescent's projections, (that is, the adolescent's personal feelings attributed to the nurse) which the nurse then perceives as the adolescent's needs. The dilemma can be seen when adolescents use aggressive, bullying tactics to intimidate the nurse into allowing them to break rules. The nurse may perceive the aggression to be anxious bluster and decides that the adolescents need sympathetic, non punitive responses to make them feel secure. An alternative however is to be frightened by the aggression and so give way to keep the peace or to gain the adolescents' approval. What is interesting is that security is not achieved by backing down nor is approval achieved by being intimidated. Security and approval are gained by firm adherence to the nurse role expected by the adolescent. Understanding the nature of the conflict does not mean that the nurse is immediately able to change behaviour, but it can give enough confidence to try it out. This does not make setting limits feel easier but the ability to do so is confirmed, giving the nurse confidence. In other words the problem is redefined, making it more manageable.

Feeling de-skilled or unskilled

Adolescents have a tremendous ability to make us feel useless and incompetent. Their challenge to society, family, authority figures and peers, which results in discovery of personal identity, shakes the identity of the recipients of the challenge. Feeling useless is common to all practitioners but is immensely strong in new and junior staff. The adolescents often pick this up and capitalise on it by checking decisions with senior, 'powerful' staff members. Intense feelings of uselessness may be related to the adolescents' view of themselves, projected onto staff members.

Dealing with these feelings results from believing a few principles:

1 Feeling useless does not mean that we are.
2 We do not need to compensate by being super-competent.
3 It is not losing face to admit our own feelings.
4 Our own feelings are useful as a guide to the adolescent's feeling of impotence.

Belief in the principles seems to free the nurse to live with these feelings whilst continuing to practice. By just continuing to practice the nurse gains respect from the adolescents, who cease to be so intensely challenging. Eventually, nurses gain confidence and use such feelings to understand adolescents, as well as to evaluate accurately their own skills.

Wanting to attack the patients

The most intense aggression directed to a patient that I have observed was by a very caring male nurse to a four-year-old. What surprised the nurse was that he actually wanted to harm a small, pathetic little boy, and this naturally made him guilty. Time after time nurses come to me to 'confess' their feelings of anger and hatred to patients. My usual response is that it comes as no surprise and is a normal reaction and in general understandable. What appears to happen is that the nurse is taken aback to find that the recipients of care do not always want it, or are not grateful. This can be demonstrated by their resisting relationships or therapy, often with verbal and physical aggression. The nurse feels rejected and is often hurt, but being bound by a professional code does not prevent frustration and pain from building up to a desire to pay the child back for hurt caused. Two things are apparent to the observer: young people however young or handicapped are not without power; and the professional codes do not forbid displeasure from being expressed. Expressing anger and frustration is necessary before they escalate to violent antipathy. Controlled statements of feelings to the young person concerned can be useful and can educate them about their effects on others. It is also useful to express these feelings to peers, and the nurse will then find that it is not just a personal affliction. Support is not limited to what the tutor or supervisor offers. Other colleagues can also provide emotional and practical support, for example, by debriefing after painful experiences.

Overattachment to one adolescent

Some nurses feel that liking a patient is the first step on the slippery slope to over-attachment. This is a problem which can cause anguish if it reflects an overall reluctance to enter relationships; it can then be a real problem which cannot be dealt with by supervision alone. I would try to steer the nurse towards personal therapy, but usually the nature of the work is such that the nurse leaves or seeks promotion as a distancing mechanism.

An alternative difficulty is to become so engrossed in one adolescent's problems that there is a failure to see the others or to work as a team member.

Jane is a course member who experienced this problem, first with a schizophrenic girl whom she felt was being neglected. The second occasion was with a boy of eight who presented to her as a baby, and very anxious; she felt that others saw him only as an odd boy and a troublemaker. Jane was allocated to both these young people and she believed herself to be the only one to fight for their rights and proper care. Through supervision, her tutor helped her to mobilise her energy to organise care plans but not to try to take over the caring. This she was in danger of doing because she antagonised other staff who perceived implied criticism of their ability to care.

The dynamics of attachment to individual young people seems due to counter-transference and to identification with some aspect of the perceived problem. I do not think that this is always detrimental because all young people need someone to believe in them, like them, and fight for their rights. It is however important that the mechanism is spotted so that one's own feelings are owned and the young people not deprived of responsibilty for their own difficulties. This achieved, energy can be directed into therapeutic interventions rather than arguing with team members or fighting all the adolescent's battles.

Antipathy towards other team members and the adolescent's family

Antipathy towards others is often couched in terms of righteous indignation at their failings compared with one's own attempts at excellence. This can be as a result of attachment to a child as in the last example, but it can be more systematic and generalised.

Antipathy to parents is common; it is as if the nurses want to save children from their families, and results from locating blame for problems in parents, who are seen as having harmed their children. Nurses perceive the child as having suffered and in need of their good parenting, so that all will be put right. This optimism is usually tempered when the adolescent is not quickly cured, but this may then be attributed to parental sabotage. Similar mechanisms are frequently at work when team members disagree and become polarised. The polarisation often occurs when a painful decision has to be made.

For example, John came to see me when at odds with other team members about the treatment of a teenager with chlorpromazine. Other professions believed that the boy was psychotic and his family frightened by his dangerous behaviour; the drug seemed to be clearly indicated. John did not 'believe' in illness, and saw the boy as lacking in good parenting and suffering developmental delay in his frustration tolerance and autonomy. John wanted to save the boy from his family and other team members. Resolving the problem was not easy and it is important to recognise basic conceptual differences between John and others. Areas of agreement were identified such as the boy's distress and his need for consistency to give him security. At the same time John tried to demonstrate his 'rightness' and to disprove the alternative view by conducting a detailed assessment. As could be predicted no clear answer was forthcoming but certain of John's points were taken up. Eventually he felt less isolated and therefore less angry with team members, but he held onto the difficulty of two intellectual viewpoints. While the boy became better John never felt easy holding onto two viewpoints; he wanted one straightforward correct solution.

Reduction of antipathy results from empathising with other points of view and other people's problems. Internal conflict is not completely resolved, and indeed if it were the energy to develop would vanish.

Desire for sameness of interventions

To count the number of times young people use 'it's not fair' to justify a grievance is probably impossible; what is interesting is that it is catching. Nurses use the argument to complain about therapeutic interventions, the off-duty rota, and not infrequently my demands as a tutor. There seems to be a myth that fairness is achieved by a uniform approach! We could however be uniformly unfair in terms of failure to consider the individual needs of others. Fairness is a difficult concept to put into practice as most people consider themselves or their patients first. I am often tempted to throw it out as a workable concept and say 'so what' when I hear the plea. Then I think again and try to look at the components of the plea to arrive at a 'fair' compromise.

> A course member devised a detailed assessment schedule for a profoundly handicapped teenage girl. The assessment was planned to demonstrate assets as well as problem behaviour. He had to work very hard to train his colleagues in new assessment techniques, even though everyone wanted the girl to have a balanced evaluation. The hurdle was crossed and the assessment was completed. The course member was then allocated another patient, also a very handicapped girl. Staff members were not satisfied with the straightforward problem checklist sheet he devised. They complained that it was not detailed enough and concentrated on problems. They then suggested a repeat of the previous girl's assessment – masochists all!

What was happening? It seems that having learnt a new and demanding technique to get it right for one girl, it was only fair to repeat the process and get it right for the next. This ignored the flaws in the first schedule, and the differences between the two girls, and the latter is particularly important.

I do not advocate throwing out all rules, but I would make a plea to vary the package we offer adolescents. It seems to make more sense to put energy into a creative flair rather than fighting for sameness. Each adolescent, and indeed each staff member, have their own needs, are at a different stage of development and have unique personalities. Most adolescents can accept changes in care that are tailored to individual needs, but nurses often get stuck with fairness and become resistant to change if there is no 'adult' around to point out the dilemma.

The problems described so far relate to the feelings and thoughts that have frequently caused nurses concern. It is now necessary to change the focus and look at two examples of situations which produce many of the feelings described, and can be the focus of hours of discussion.

Suspending or discharging an adolescent

It can happen that a patient is discharged or suspended from the unit for breaking major rules, resistance to therapy, stretching staff beyond reasonable limits or not abiding by a contract for care. The latter is often not a contract as such but a staff decision about the direction of care. In principle I accept the need for discharge or suspension which can give therapeutic leverage, or be a statement about the unit's and adolescent's inability to work together for change. I find it difficult to accept that an adolescent can be discharged or suspended for the same reasons as those for which he was admitted. This most frequently happens with adolescents admitted for conduct problems that parents and society cannot deal with.

The dynamics of precipitate ejection include the frustration of optimistic hopes for change; feeling rejected by someone we want to care for; and mounting anger when earlier difficulties are ignored or discounted by other team members. It seems that the weight of this is projected onto the adolescent; it is his fault and consequently he becomes the scapegoat. Occasionally despair about lack of success becomes a countertransference issue, and we collude with the child's despair. In the discussions about these two courses of action a lone voice may be heard arguing for continued efforts. The owner of this voice often becomes identified with the scapegoat position, and this is reinforced by fighting alone against a tide of opinion which seeks conformity. My belief in the unconscious at work during these discussions is confirmed by trying to remember the exact reasons for the action some time later. I can often remember events but the emotion has gone, and the adolescent's behaviour seems to me nothing out of the ordinary and often better than that of other patients not discharged.

As course tutor I try to examine the feelings of nurses in situations which generate heat. Looking at feelings is usually more profitable than examining the reasons for the action. I have been so angry as the lone voice that it has been difficult to avoid tears or verbal abuse. At other times I have been angry at being made to feel guilty by the lone voice, and consequently renewed the fight to oppose them. By exploring feelings some of the worst, excesses of team fighting can be avoided. Sometimes the proposal to eject the adolescent will be refused; but should it stand we are, I hope, not so punitive as to completely close the door on further contracts for care. The aim I would identify is that team relationships and the adolescent in question should not be permanently scarred by the excesses of unconscious mechanisms.

Non-compliance

This becomes a problem when nurses identify it as the patient's problem. Rarely do adolescents see non-compliance as their problem, and indeed their refusal to comply is perceived as the problem of nurses who demand obedience. This tautology describes a circular and interactional dilemma, and my reason for drawing attention to it is that it can cause great distress. A nurse recently presented me with an assessment sheet in which nurses had to tick the following categories:

ready compliance with ward expectations

reluctant compliance

refusal to comply

In this instance compliance turned out to be related to going to meals and the problem could be redefined as reluctance to eat. The redefinition gives the problem back to the patient and leads to different management interventions.

It is possible to describe non-compliance in terms of nurses internalising the adolescents' rebelliousness and then defining their feelings as the patients' problem. By doing this they make interventions difficult, because people rarely comply totally with the wishes of others even when there is a strong relationship and a desire to please. The problem is more accurately put as one of defining a level of acceptable behaviour with defined limits. To miss this point is likely to lead to failure and unfortunately is perceived as a failure of nursing or the adolescent's failure to change. In other words a recipe for disaster. The remedy is to examine patient problems in the light of how we feel towards both patient and problem. Acknowledging personal dilemmas allows precise definition of patient problems and helps to keep them located with the patient. This makes evaluation of care and patient change both more realistic and more useful.

Strategies to Assist Learning

In this account of some common problems my approach to teaching may have become obvious, but I will conclude with a short description of strategies that I have employed to help myself and I hope others. Strategies which facilitate learning and maintenance of good practice are not always comfortable. This point if remembered can avoid participants giving up.

The most common strategy is talking, in groups and in one to one sessions with a supervisor. Group discussion can be formal topic discussions in an educational sense (Abercrombie 1970) or they can be formal groups. The latter are often called staff support groups, a most glaring misnomer implying bolstering people and fostering agreement. These groups are most useful and while they can offer the comfort of shared experience, should also address themselves to the feelings of participants, which are often painful and diverse. The group will not then be comfortable. There is a danger that the pain will be attributed to the group or the group leader, and both can be scapegoated. This will result in avoidance of the group, isolation of the leader, attacking the leader and possibly ejecting the leader. A most important part of staff groups is in learning to own personal difficulty, and then working with others to resolve the conflict. Acceptance of this principle allows groups to be supportive and useful, indeed they can be a most important aspect of work on a unit or on a course. This statement is validated by evaluative statements of the course members during five years who ranked their groupwork as being the most significant experience offered.

Talking one to one with a supervisor is also an important way of understanding and exploring personal beliefs and behaviour as well as allowing time for individual theoretical discussion. This experience attaches value to individuals and helps them to take themselves and their learning seriously. To do this the sessions should be directed by the learners, who bring for discussion what is important to themselves. This assists motivation for change and promotes good teacher – learner relationships.

Other strategies involve action as well as talking. Of these, observed practice with feedback is the most useful way to enhance skill and change behaviour. There must be trust between practitioner and supervisor, and the experience allows immediate trying out of suggestions. Success then reinforces desirable behaviour and it is possible to give praise for something seen rather than reported. This praise is usually acknowledged as being more valid because it avoids the vagaries of the learner's memory. Other ways of offering this type of supervision involve using video records or role play practice with peers. Both are very useful, and role play has another dimension, it can be fun; especially when participants exaggerate problems, facing the teacher with the problem of keeping a straight face.

Sculpting is a non-verbal technique which highlights the importance of positional relationships. Without a word participants experience the emotions which may result from putting themselves in other peoples shoes. The latter occurs also in role play using role-reversal.

Developing empathy with the experience of others is a vital part of learning for those whose job involves relationships. By empathising one can judge personal response and make it as useful as possible for the recipient. Both sculpting and role play are action techniques which affect the emotions of participants. By exploring these light is thrown on relationship and interactional issues, and these feelings, linked to cognitive work, will bring about learning in a powerful way. The intense experience has the power to change attitudes as well as to teach behavioural skills.

Conclusions

Support, supervision and training are the components of useful learning experience. We need to feel approval from and trust in the teacher, and these can be labelled support. Supervision related to actual practice helps learning because it is relevant to the work and provides space to link theoretical concepts with action. It is also a way of guiding skill development without waiting for solitary trial and error. Training implies that we will not be left to flounder in a sea of ignorance and fear.

All practitioners are also learners; whilst I teach and supervise others it is well known that I seek supervision and ideas from others. I also learn from learners, a practice discovered by a course member given the job of teaching a junior student. He discovered that efforts to help the student consolidated and stretched his own knowledge and skill. The reciprocal nature of the student-teacher relationship compares with the patient-nurse relationship. We learn from all experiences; whatever the patient does to or for us is a potentially enhancing experience. This is not always immediately evident, indeed I can think of some adolescents who aided learning I could have done without! I have however learnt the value of exploring all these aspects of practice, the relationships, feelings, skills and theory, in an attempt to improve personal performance and facilitate change in patients. It is important to recognise that support, supervision and training are integral components of a whole learning experience and not ends in themselves.

References and Further Reading

Abercrombie M L J (1970) *Aims and Techniques of Group Teaching.* Society for research into Higher Education

Gagne R M (1970) *The Conditions of Learning.* New York: Rinehart & Winston

Blatner H A (1973) *Acting-in Practical Application of Psycho-dramatic Methods.* Springer

Bruner J S (1972) *The Relevance of Education.* Harmondsworth: Penguin Books

Rogers C R (1967) *"On Becoming a Person": A Therapist's view of Psychotherapy.* London: Constable

Wilkinson T R (1983) *Child and Adolescent Psychiatric Nursing.* Oxford: Blackwell Scientific Publications

The Adolescent Unit
Edited by Derek Steinberg
© 1986 D. Steinberg

17 The Staff Group

John Foskett

Biographical note: see chapter 14

It is ten o'clock on a Friday morning. I am seated in a chair opposite the clock on the wall. The room is bright with sunlight pouring in through the large windows catching the colours of the brightly painted pictures and posters. Some chairs in a circle at one end, together with a few empty coffee cups are reminders of yesterday's meetings and a sign of unreadiness for today's. From the corridor outside comes the sound of people talking. In they come, a group of young men and women, some dressed casually and some extravagantly, occupied and excited by their conversation. They push the chairs back, dropping into them and falling silent as they do. Someone arrives breathless and glancing at the clock sits down with sigh of relief. He's not as late as he thought. Others come in, one with a cup of coffee and a jocular greeting 'I'm not apologising'; others laugh. Yet another slips in hesitatingly, and asks if an empty chair belongs to anyone else. The door is finally shut and the group becomes still and silent; most are looking at the floor. After some minutes the hesitant member looks enquiringly around and then says 'Can anyone tell me what this group is for?'

Heads rise, eyes catch and breaths are held. Someone smiles knowingly as if wondering 'Who's going to explain?', and the unvoiced question passes silently around the group. I wonder what the reply is going to be this time. 'I was just thinking the same'; or 'That is the question we all keep asking'; 'We expect that of new people'; or 'Hasn't anyone explained that to you yet?' In these ways, the questioner may be sympathised with, educated, accused, appointed a leader, applauded for her bravery, or ignored, for sometimes nothing is said at all and the group returns to concentrating upon the floor.

'What are staff groups for?' is a proper and important question. Groups like this one are found in most psychiatric hospitals and clinics. They appear on the weekly timetable, form a part of the training programmes of most health care disciplines and have a special place in the mythology of good staff development. What is more, they are an expense to the Health Service. Keeping some twenty members of staff of all grades in one room for an hour each week demands some assessment of cost effectiveness.

'What are staff groups for?' matters in another way. It is reasonable to assume that human beings function more effectively and usefully if they know what they

169

are doing. And it is the aim of this chapter to help staff, both experienced and inexperienced in groups, to clarify for themselves what their staff group is for; or at least to see what it could be for, and to consider what needs to be done if such a group is to help staff function effectively.

However, before embarking upon a discussion of these matters, it may help to clarify why there is a mystery about such groups in the first place. Other meetings of health care professionals, like ward rounds or case discussions, are taken for granted, but these have agendas, specific procedures that are more or less adhered to: they review past decisions and actions, draw together conclusions, and make fresh decisions. Although there may be some baffling and confusing aspects to these meetings it is possible to see what they are for. So why is there a mystery surrounding staff groups, a mystery which is not dispelled by calling them 'support' or 'sensitivity' groups? Central to the mystery is the nature of the groups themselves. They are not primarily about achieving some particular end or reaching some predetermined goal – they are more literally about themselves, an end in themselves. They provide staff with an opportunity to pause in their work and take some stock of what they are doing; to reflect upon their experience of striving after 'ends' and 'goals', to see where their efforts have got them and to find out the effect it has had upon them. It is in that sense that the group is mysterious: no-one knows beforehand what the meeting will reveal. At the end it may not be much clearer either, but the attempt has been made to pause and reflect upon the experience of work as it has been and is influencing the staff who gather today, and who in some way represent all who could or might attend.

If we return to the staff group whose beginning we recorded, perhaps it will be easier to see what already has been revealed about the group's purpose. It has brought the staff of this unit together, in one place and at one time. Individuals and whole professions have come from different places, physically different, the nurses from the ward, the teachers from the school and the secretary from her office; and they are also personally and professionally different. A nurse from a frightening interaction with a patient; the teachers from a meeting to replan their timetable; a doctor from his struggle to complete a summary on one of the patients; a social worker brooding over a difficult family meeting last night; and the occupational therapist torn between his need to be at both this and his own department's meeting. The group collects them all together and so by its very existence is a reminder that though they come from different places with different occupations and pre-occupations, they are involved in a common enterprise.

This group began as though that were not the case; individuals were preoccupied with their own thoughts. They looked at the floor, and were reluctant even to make eye contact. In contrast, last week's group began in a much more animated way with everyone discussing arrangements for a unit outing. So the behaviour of the group, whatever it is, will tell us something of the unit's emotional climate. Today it is withdrawn, preoccupied and separate. But more than that has been revealed already. One group of nurses arrived bringing with them a sense of excitement and interest, a little like parents who have got their children off to school and are now free to relate to one another. A doctor thought he was late, and someone else wasn't going to apologise for bringing their coffee, a tangible symbol of sustenance, with them. Yet another, the person to speak first, conveyed her unease. All have demonstrated something about themselves, something about themselves in relation to this unit, and so something about the unit. By the group's existence and its beginning we, that is those who are present, have the chance to collect ourselves, to witness and experience the bits and pieces of behaviour, to get a feel for the unit today.

As leader or facilitator to the group, I, too, have given a message by my behaviour. By arriving on time and sitting opposite the clock I am saying something about one of the important limits of the group. It is for an hour, and this hour each week, it has a beginning and an end which I always observe. So one aspect of my leadership is related to the boundaries or limits of the group, but in another sense I am obviously not a leader. I do not explain what this group is for when the question is asked, and so I help to demonstrate the difference between this group and other meetings where the leader behaves more like a chairman. I try to show my readiness to address the mystery of the group: to await rather than provoke revelation, to begin to piece together the events, the behaviour, the words and most of all the feelings of the group as it proceeds, to collect and store away the kind of observations I have already mentioned and compare them with my own feelings. Already I have felt animosity, amusement, embarrassment and, like everyone else, I was quickly absorbed by my own thoughts and distracted from thinking about the meeting itself. If I had been clearer in my own mind about any of this, then I might have spoken tentatively about what I perceived or felt. Perhaps it was the sense of the group slipping away which activated the newest member and forced out the question 'Could someone tell me what this group is for?'

Certainly, it led the members of the group to look at one another for the first time. The familiar question reminded them of what they have in common and, ironically, of how the newest recruit had already joined them in their mystery. As was mentioned, the response to the question carries the process of the group a stage further, revealing something more of what the silence was about. A senior member of staff begins to explain the purpose of the group, and so to give a lead and guidance to the newcomer. One might guess that issues about leadership and guidance, or the relationship between leaders and led is of some importance to the unit. On another similar occasion, nothing was said and the questioner was left puzzled and embarrassed, perhaps demonstrating a frustration on the part of others with all the changes, and a reluctance to acknowledge the arrival of new people, or perhaps there was some other issue of such importance to the group that it would not have its silent deliberation interrupted. Whatever the behaviour of the group, it will in one way or another begin to tell its story; each moment, every response or silence, will leave its mark. Like a jigsaw puzzle gradually taking shape, a picture will begin to appear; some pieces will fit and others will not.

Today it is the issue of leaders and led. It emerges in different forms which reflect the way the issue impinges upon different people. The teachers are expecting a new senior member of staff and they have mixed feelings about it, missing their former colleague and being anxious about their new one. The nurses are trying to institute a fresh daily programme on the ward and are being frustrated in turn by the patients, other professions and their own administration. The unit as a whole has to decide whether or not to invite the patients' parents to a forthcoming concert. Some will come and others will not, the patients are divided about it, and the staff are anxious about how they will cope on the night itself. All touch upon the real difficulties of leading and being led. I find myself drawn into this discussion and begin to add my suggestions and comments like any other member of the group. Before long I, too, am taking a lead, which appears to be as difficult to follow as anyone else's. Puzzled and frustrated, I stop. Then one of the nursing assistants says that she cannot contain herself any longer. She is fed up with the way some of her colleagues (her seniors who are not present) left her to do a difficult job, and, after she failed, were so quick with helpful explanations. The outburst relieves the tension much in the same way that the original question eased and united the group. It is as if everyone can recognise and share the frustration of the nursing assistant. In fact, it prompts others to tell their own stories of the gap between knowledge and experience, saying and doing. Knowing about something and yet not being able to use or apply that knowledge satisfactorily touches some of the central issues for the unit. The majority of staff are here to learn as well as to care and to treat, and their learning is hewn out of the interaction between experience and knowledge, thoughts and actions. It is hard-won learning that never remains static and is always tested by the next event.

This is also a reflection of a central issue of adolescence. The patients are struggling, too, with the interaction of knowledge and experience. In one way or another, their struggle is the result of some breakdown in that interaction. So they bring their sense of frustration, resentment and despair and, by projection, hand much of it over to their carers and therapists. Rarely do they voice it, but nevertheless they seem to be saying: 'Don't tell us about growing up, don't explain it. Show us yourselves how you manage the really difficult bits. Stay with us when the going gets tough and then let us see how you cope when life is as crazy and impossible as we find it. If you can hang on then, well, perhaps there is some hope for us after all. But we need more than anything else to test your stamina, your capacity not just to know about what's wrong, but actually to bear it'.

At this meeting the group demonstrated something of the way in which it does hold and contain the anxiety it has been given. At first it bears its feelings in silence, and then gradually and tentatively it brings them out into the open. Often the group's mouthpiece is a new or junior member of staff, those who are not expected to know everything and therefore have less to lose than their more experienced colleagues. The nursing assistant spoke for the group as well as herself in her outburst. Once the lid covering difficult and unexpressed emotions is lifted the group may well need quickly to defend itself again. This is done when the outburst is ignored and the unlucky individual is left to cope with all the feelings by herself, or when someone begins to explain what happened and justify their actions. Either move can have the effect of repressing the feelings once again or the opposite, adding more fuel to the fire. Whatever happens there is a sense in which the staff begin to address the emotion-laden issues, this time the one of leading and being led, in the relative security of their own meeting. Their strengths and weaknesses are tested among themselves as a preparation for the work they are about to begin again.

The hour is up and the group disperses, individuals taking away their own thoughts and feelings, but now from a common pool of shared experience. No-one will have fully digested the significance of what has been happening, but nevertheless a lot has been chewed over and so can begin to feed and nourish the unit's system. From the original sense of separateness and weighty preoccupation, the staff have struggled first to collect themselves together and then slowly to acknowledge what is holding them apart. They have identified the issue which most needs their attention, and by addressing it in here they have made it that much easier to attend to it out there.

Of course, much of the mystery remains, for no-one has reached any decision and no plans have been publicly made. Rather, as the metaphor above suggests, there has been much food for thought, exploration of feelings and attention to the staff's personal and professional interface. They have swallowed a great deal, chewed on some, and now begin to digest it. Just as we cannot see how food keeps us alive, so it is difficult to see how the group enlivens this unit. But it is unlikely that teaching sessions, either of the patients or the staff, will be unaffected by it in the week ahead. Perhaps, too, the burdens of difficult tasks will be redistributed a little, the patients made more aware of the unit's stamina, and of the staff's ability to carry the adolescents' projections. The staff themselves may feel that much less alone, and more in the company of colleagues who are struggling with the same things. Maybe not much will change and next Friday will reveal yet more resentment and frustration. Once again, the staff will have to collect themselves together, to find the energy and confidence to dig more deeply and more honestly in order to unearth whatever it is that is getting in their way.

The metaphor of a digestive system illustrates well both the nature and the purpose of a staff group. It takes in whatever the unit brings to it, it then works to digest what it has swallowed to feed the various parts with the food they need, and to alert the whole body or system to the needs which are not being met. Like all digestive systems, the group can function more or less well. It can be deprived of food, it can reject what it has swallowed, it can digest some things and not others, and so defend itself against whatever tastes bad. Over a period of time the digestive patterns will become clearer, and the unit more able to read and understand the signs and symptoms. In order to do this, it helps if the unit can share a common theory, language, or perspective about groups. The particular theory probably matters less than the fact that it is a shared one, not shared in the sense that everyone understands it in details, but that it is seen to help make sense of the jumbled experience we have already recorded. Inevitably the group's leader has to embody this theory, and should be chosen on the basis that he works with a theory which the unit as a whole finds compatible and understandable. The theory with which I work is based upon that of Bion (1968); others have found the principles of Foulkes & Anthony (1957), Balint (1957) and systems theory (Skynner 1976) helpful.

Group Processes

Bion (1968) studied groups firstly in a psychiatric hospital, and then in psycho-therapeutic groups, but the principles of his theory have been applied to groups in industry and commerce (Rice, 1963), education (Bazalgette 1971), religion (Reed 1979), and more widely in the health and social services (Menzies 1979; Bridger 1978). Most of us are aware of the complicated nature of groups; often what they do is different from what they say they are doing, and their hidden agendas can be more influential than their open ones. In order to understand what he found to be so confusing about groups Bion hypothesised that groups function on two, often unconnected, levels.

At the *work or task level* people meet to perform some activity: to sell goods, score goals, manufacture something or navigate at sea. Staff in the unit can meet with clear goals, as in a case discussion or teaching session. Bion saw that groups also met to do something for themselves which was not necessarily related to their work. At times he noticed that the group's tasks were forgotten as individuals directed all their energies towards their own preservation and maintenance, as if a ship is about to sink. Often the threat isn't clear, although the group acts as if it is; the group acts 'as if' the work task is for the moment irrelevant and responds instead to an unconscious *basic assumption*, which is the other level. Bion, starting from his own experience as the member of a tank crew in the First World War, believed that groups behave this way to preserve themselves from an unconscious threat.

The group described earlier began in silence; at the task level this is a reasonable way to begin, allowing members to collect themselves and to consider what has been happening to them. At the second level, however, it may be a sign of resistance to getting on with the business. The question, 'What is the group for?' is directed to the task, but could be an alarm signal too. In fact, it led to one of the three types of behaviour Bion identified as *basic assumption* or *second level* activity; *pairing*, the questioner and a senior member of staff becoming engaged in conversation as teacher and pupil. The other patterns of behaviour Bion described were *dependency* (eg. unrealistic dependence on people, theories, events or ideas – 'all will be well when so and so returns from holiday') and *fight and flight* (arguing or withdrawing pointlessly; in all institutions there are bad objects to attack or run away from). Fight or flight is a natural defence against the clash of opposites: can elation about success be tolerated beside despair about failure? Will one not spoil the other?

Bion believed that basic assumption activity – dependence, pairing, and fight and flight – are always present though often dormant in groups and organisations, and that when the group's or organisation's first-level task is demanding, more and more of its energy and resources are devoted to second level activity unless care is taken to recognise it, to identify the threat and address it directly.

Sometimes, if members of a group can be helped to recall what they were feeling and thinking about in a silence, they can identify what the threat is about. For instance, coming together as a staff group is worrying in at least three different ways. It can be worrying personally: most of us feel safer on our own familiar ground, and what we encounter in a shared space can exaggerate or ease our personal anxiety. It can be worrying professionally: most of us feel more secure when among a group who share the same opportunities and problems. Who or which group is best at the job can be a persecuting preoccupation, just as can the feeling of envy for what others achieve. The third kind of anxiety, the tensions and problems of patients, projected on to staff, is the most difficult to detect. Being the object and carrier of other people's projections is complex, and one of the most difficult and yet most important parts of the unit's work. Through it, the staff bear some of the distress which their patients are too weak or sick to carry, and also demonstrate how burdens are carried, and how patients can gradually resume responsibility for them. The staff will often drop some of these 'burdens' on each other's toes, in order to reach this kind of anxiety and get it more equally distributed.

So the silence of the group may have been about any or all of these kinds of anxiety. The meeting provides the staff with the chance to explore and separate out their feelings and redistribute their weight more equally. When this is too much or too difficult to do, the group will adopt basic assumption activity, like the pairing already mentioned, by dependency, or by fight and flight. Pairing, in particular, is often related to issues around sexuality, creativity and potency, key concerns in an adolescent unit, and ones which fit well with family dynamics, which is also a recurring theme in staff groups.

Establishing Staff Groups

Staff groups are organised for a variety of reasons more or less related to the task (level one) and unconscious needs (level two) of the organisation. To be most effective in the terms set out above, groups require the active but not uncritical support of everyone, and particularly of those responsible for the unit's work. The initiative for starting can come from anywhere or anyone, but it must then be understood and accepted at all levels within the unit. This can often take a considerable time, but it is important for group enthusiasts to be patient, and group critics to have their say, or the group is likely to be frustrating and unproductive.

The following guidelines need to be borne in mind before starting.

1 All the staff of the unit should be consulted about the possibility of having a group. This is best done through the normal channels; if these do not exist, they must be created first. The more thoroughly and extensive the consultation the better

it will be for the group. Administrative, domestic and clerical staff should be included, as well as the health care professions.

2 The senior members of all the disciplines who have ultimate responsibility for the work of the unit, and those in line management between them and the unit staff; the medical executive committee; hospital administration; social work, psychology, occupational therapy, education and chaplaincy departments; these should all be informed and their reactions noted.

3 Following consultation, those responsible can decide whether or not to start a group, possibly on an experimental basis with a review built in.

4 A group contract should be drawn up to include the following:

(a) *The Time and the Place of the group.* This should be agreed upon so that the maximum number of staff of all levels can attend. The hierarchies of all disciplines and teaching establishments should be contacted to ensure that the group clashes as little as possible with other staff commitments, and that whenever these have to be altered the group is not overlooked.

(b) *The expectations* should be clarified. For instance, that all who are on duty should attend, and that regular attendance is expected. Those who cannot attend every week should nevertheless attend regularly, and apologies for non-attendance should be made in advance. A rota of all staff should be set up to provide patient care while the group meets.

(c) *The Purpose of the Group* can be expressed in a simple statement, eg. 'A group for staff to share their experience of working on the unit, and the effect of that work upon themselves and one another.'

(d) *The Confidentiality* of the group is essential. Everyone has an equal right to speak or to remain silent and should speak as far as possible for themselves and not for others. Whatever is discussed in any one meeting can be brought up in subsequent meetings, but nothing will be directly spoken about outside the meetings, unless the group decides that this needs to be done for a particular reason.

(e) *Copies of the Contract* should be given to all staff members on appointment, and the contract itself reviewed by the whole group at regular intervals.

(f) *A group leader or facilitator* should be appointed and given a contract.

Appointment of a group leader or facilitator

Units often prefer to start a staff group without a leader, or with one of their number as the appointed facilitator. It is more than likely that some members of staff will have the knowledge and expertise to lead, and some staff groups experiment with a rotational leadership. These alternatives seem to me to evade the important issue of the group trusting themselves sufficiently to trust the help of someone not of their number; helping professions are notoriously reticent in seeking help for themselves.

Ideally the leader should be skilled in some form of group work (group therapy, analysis, dynamics or relations), and should be institutionally as separate from the unit as possible. Employing and therefore paying someone from another institution is best. Perhaps a more realistic alternative is to invite someone from another department or unit within the same hospital or clinic. Some institutions (like The Tavistock Clinic) are now training consultants, and it is possible to invite one of their students to act as leader. Leaders will come from different personal and professional backgrounds, which will prejudice them (and the members of the group) in one way or another. This should be openly acknowledged and explored at the beginning of the group and at regular intervals for the sake of new members. In my experience, leaders can be manipulated into their professional and personal prejudices when the group is confronting its most stressful issues. When this happens, leaders with a background in psychotherapy are generally to be found doing therapy, social workers social working, nurses nursing, and chaplains preaching, instead of helping with the task. They do this to the obvious relief of everyone but with very little effect upon the issue itself. It is helpful if the leader and the group get used to this behaviour so that they can recognise it for what it is. There may well be a case here for health service groups employing leaders from industry or education, who are less likely to become embroiled in the evasions common to those who work in health or social services. Caplan (1970) and Steinberg and Yule (1985) have made important contributions to our understanding of the role of the facilitator in consultative work of this kind, and of the importance of the way in which the work is done.

References and Further Reading

Balint M (1968) *The Doctor, the Patient and the Illness*. London: Pitman

Bazalgette J (1971) *Freedom, Authority and the Young Adult*. London: Pitman

Bion W R (1968) *Experiences in Groups*, London: Tavistock

Bridger H (1978) The increasing relevance of group processes and changing values for understanding and coping with stress at work. In C L Cooper & R Payne (eds) *Stress at Work*. Chichester: Wiley

Caplan G (1970) *The Theory and Practice of Mental Health Consultation*, New York: Basic Books

De Board R (1978) *The Psychoanalysis of Organisations*. London: Tavistock

Foulkes S H, Anthony E J (1957) *Group Psychotherapy, the Psychodynamic Approach*. Harmondsworth: Penguin Books

Kolb D A, Rubin I M & McItyre J M (1974) *Organisational Psychology: An Experiential Approach*. New Jersey: Prentice Hall

Menzies I E P (1970) *The Functioning of Social Systems as a Defence against Anxiety*. London: Tavistock Institute of Human Relations

Reed B (1978) *The Dynamics of Religion: Process and Movement in Christian Churches*. London: Darton, Longman & Todd

Rice A K (1963) *The Enterprise and its Environment*. London: Tavistock

Rioch M J (1970) The work of Wilfred Bion on groups. *Psychiatry*, **33**, 56-66

Skynner A C R (1975) The large group in training. In L C Kreeger (ed) *The Large Group Dynamics and Therapy, Constable*, London

Skynner A C R (1976). *One Flesh: Separate Persons*. London: Constable

Steinberg D & Yule W (1985) Consultative work. In M Rutter & L Hersov (eds) *Child and Adolescent Psychiatry: Modern Approaches*. Oxford: Blackwell

Winnicott D W (1974) *Playing and Reality*. Harmondsworth: Penguin Books, pp. 169-173

The Adolescent Unit
Edited by Derek Steinberg
© 1986 D. Steinberg

18 Aspects of Leadership

John Lampen

When I went to Oxford to study Greek and Roman history and philosophy, after a period of army service, I had no idea what work I would like to take up. Two things pointed me towards a decision: the first was a series of summer camps with Borstal boys, organised by my college; and the second was the press report of a riot in an approved school and the subsequent enquiry, which led me to feel that if such schools were run in the way described, the sooner something was done to change this the better. I applied to take a Diploma in Education, and, a year later in the summer of 1962, newly married, I joined the staff not of an approved school but of Shotton Hall, one of the pioneering schools for adolescent maladjusted boys. The founder and Principal was Fred Lennhoff OBE, a refugee from Nazi Germany, a friend of Alfred Adler, a volatile, uniquely gifted and unforgettable leader and guide. His insight, originality and creativity made him marvellous to work with and learn from, while the contradictions in his personality also made it very stressful at times. Ten years later, having set up a charitable trust to ensure the continuation of the school, he passed its leadership on to me, and died little over two years later.

This was the introduction and training for my work, apart from a part-time psychotherapy course some years later; to me it feels enough, not least because it has given me the belief that one learns on and through the job and that this process is never finished. I am glad, too, to have always worked in a setting where education and treatment shaded into one another and where there were no specialist workers fighting (or even negotiating) to establish the priority of their own departments.

Schools for maladjusted children have come in for considerable criticism recently. In the case of Shotton Hall, the leavers over a five-year period have been followed up in great detail, and I am content to await this verdict on our work. In general, such schools offer provision for boys and girls who are causing severe anxiety to others at home, at school, or in the local community; the provision is for a longer period than most adolescent psychiatric units, and has a defined purpose for the youngster and a regular alternation of term and holiday which contrasts with children's or community homes. Moreover, the placing authority (where financial considerations permit) can choose between a large number of differing styles of regime instead of having to use one of a very few local institutions. Lastly, the school for maladjusted children provides an integrated experience and, particularly if independent, has the freedom to develop its approach experimentally. There is no justification for any individual school except the quality of its work; but I think there is a good case for those who have to make decisions about helping damaged, deprived and disturbed young people having not only a number of treatment settings to choose from, but also different types of setting.

179

During my work at Shotton Hall, I grew interested in questions of stress and conflict and their resolution in the wider community. After twenty years there, my wife and I decided we were ready for a change, so we have moved to Londonderry to learn new skills and face new challenges.

———◆———

The Leader's Dilemma

A boy of thirteen ran into my room one day, screaming and crying. When he had calmed down enough to be able to speak, he claimed that our newest teacher had attacked him. Knowing the amount of provocation this boy could offer, I tried to learn what happened before as well as during the tussle, but he kept screaming 'What are you going to do about him?' While this was happening the teacher came in, obviously still in the grip of his anger with the boy, who immediately fell into a glowering silence. I asked the boy to tell us both what had happened. He started: the teacher almost at once tried to correct him, and I had to ask him to wait. The boy began again, a little more frankly. The story was predictable – the boy's unease with a new teacher had led him to push his provocation beyond reasonable bounds; the teacher, also uneasy in a new situation, had over-reacted; both of them were now frightened and guilty at the strength of that reaction.

What did they now want from me? Each of them might have said 'Justice', but they would have meant something very different by it. Beyond the boy's belief that he deserved some recompense for a physical assault lay a more basic fear: he knew he had gone too far, but he knew he was liable to go too far again, so how could he be safe from the violence he evoked in this man? If I responded to the teacher's pressure to put him in the wrong, I offered him no safety; but he was not really better off if I said that the teacher was to blame, for he knew the teacher would not accept that verdict and would resent him as the cause of his reprimand. The teacher believed that justice would consist in my support for his wish to have an orderly class (and who came blame him?), but beyond this lay a forlorn hope that, from a distance, I could exert enough influence on events in his classroom to save him from another loss of self-control.

My dilemma as leader starts from the fact that I am responsible for the boy's actual safety and feeling of security; if I fail him, he is justified in running away or ringing the police next time, but at present he has faith in me. I have a more fundamental duty to the boy than to the teacher. But I am also responsible for ensuring that the teaching of the school gets done, and that those who want to learn are not disrupted by those who don't. I must not unthinkingly put this boy's interests before those of the group. And the problem is complicated by the fact that this teacher has real immediate needs: the boy has been in scrapes of all kinds before, and somehow survives; but if I fail the teacher, he is justified in trying to organise his colleagues in a protest, or giving in his notice, or continuing to work as a disillusioned hack who sees no reason to give of his best. And both of them have defined already (or, in my view, misdefined) the type of action by me which will meet the claims of 'justice'.

I should point out here that in the world as we have it, some one person will have my responsibility. I will refer briefly to collective leadership later; but if there is a collective or delegated responsibility, or a school or unit 'meeting' or 'court' to handle such matters, this will be because a designated person in my position believes it is right to delegate his authority in one of these ways. Ultimately the decision what to do about this incident, or about all such incidents, depends on how one person interprets the ethos of the setting. He may not have created the ethos; it may have come from a whole treatment philosophy, or from the beliefs of a committee, or some other outside authority. But the decision by this one person at this point affects what both staff and inmates take that ethos to mean.

So I may decide that it is ultimately in the boy's interest, as well as everyone else's, to see that there is no 'messing about' in class. Or I may give priority to impressing on the teacher that, whatever the provocation, this is a place where staff do not hit children. I may emphasise that here we believe that such conflicts are everyone's concern, and are only sorted out when everyone is present. Or I may try what mediating skills I have to get these two people to understand and sympathise with one another's difficulties, and make a joint agreement about how to help one another in future, which is what I did on this occasion. It is not that one of these solutions is obviously the right one; each of them has some deficiencies and might well need some follow-up. For instance, if there is to be a group meeting, the teacher will almost certainly need help with his feelings about being 'put on a par' with this boy, and 'judged by other boys'. But, by his choices, the leader establishes or fails to establish the character and effectiveness of his little world.

Is a Leader Necessary?

This question is seldom asked, since most of us grow up and are educated within hierarchical systems. Indeed, when there are participatory systems, it has usually needed one dynamic individual to conceptualise, organise and defend them, whether in an institution or society as a whole; and such people may not find it easy to delegate their authority or lay it down. Maxwell Jones (1976) suggests that the therapeutic community may need charismatic leadership at the start, but it can be transformed by way of a stage of multiple leadership into a self-sufficient, self-regulating community. We do not yet know enough about the 'life-cycle' of institutions to evaluate this; but the 'messianic' character of the community implicit in Jones' thesis has been criticised by Robert Hobson (in Hinshelwood & Manning 1979):

A democracy depends upon power; certainly the power of love and of respect but in the last resort upon coercion. That is a failure. But, to me, it seems to be a fact. In our unit, we attempt to make it explicit, not pretend that it is not so. If need be (but only as a last resort) I decide, as openly as possible, attempting to avoid subtly concealed pressure. But I hope that I listen to everyone. Really listen – deep in my middle.

Since 1945 we have become aware, as perhaps no previous generation has done, of how social class, official status, and political, economic and military strength can be exploited for personal advantage. This has been used not only to attack the concept of leadership, but also to attach a generalised feeling of guilt to the possession of power. (This may not be altogether a bad thing, particularly for workers with young people, if it increases their self-awareness.) But it makes it necessary to reaffirm that it is the *exploitation*, not the *possession*, of authority which is wrong. The leader, as Jesus of Nazareth saw clearly, should be a servant:

> You call me 'Master' and 'Lord', and rightly so, for that is what I am. Then if I, your Lord and Master, have washed your feet, you also ought to wash one another's feet. I have set you an example.

The leader is generally expected to serve the organisation in the following ways:
 (i)   maintain its viability and life-support systems;
 (ii) define, or at least interpret, the ethos and tasks of the organisation;
 (iii) establish its external boundary, and monitor crossings of the boundary;
 (iv) establish what internal boundaries are needed, how tasks are to be subdivided and power delegated;
 (v)   accept what is projected on to authority-figures from those inside and outside the organisation, and find ways to manage this.

The first of these may be managed by an outside body, the local authority or a parent hospital; or it may be a delegated task within the institution. The second, third and fourth might evolve from processes of consultation and participation within the institution as a community; and if this is done, the projections will be diffused among the members (helpers and helped) within the community and certain figures or bodies outside it. They will then be less threatening; but is collective leadership really feasible? Before thinking about this, I must make it clearer what is meant by external and internal boundaries, and look at some vital functions of leadership.

The external boundary

D W Winnicott (1974) drew attention to the complex relationship between playing and psychotherapy, and the fact that both have to happen in a place which is neither inside nor outside the individual. The treatment setting provides a physical image of this space where things can happen; and the *boundary*, like a wall round a playground, is whatever makes it safe for things to happen there. The person in charge is on the boundary, facing inwards and outwards.

Looking inwards, he says 'This is what the world expects of us. This is what we have been set up and funded to do. This is the kind of procedure we can employ without outside interference, that is not. If such-and-such happens, I will not be able to protect us from outside intervention. These events in the world outside will make a difference to how we do our job; those events will not . . .'

Looking outwards, he says 'This is the need you have asked us to meet, and these are the methods we believe will meet this need. Here is an area where we know you must dictate to us, and here is another where we need your help; but in this other area, we must have the right to make our own decisions. If you do not allow us such-and-such resources, we cannot do what you want from us . . .' and so on.

I suspect that most people in charge are temperamentally happier with one of these stances or the other; and one might expect the head who prefers interpreting the needs of the establishment to the world outside to run a more idiosyncratic, possibly radical, regime while his counterpart adopts a more traditional medical or educational model. But both of them have to encounter pressure from each direction, sometimes from both at once. One example of this is when inmates cause difficulties outside the establishment.

On my very first day as headmaster at Shotton Hall, three boys under 18 bought drink in Shrewsbury, drank too much, and were sick on the bus coming back. Talking to our local police, with whom we had good relations, I found they were not keen on prosecuting the boys, but needed to do so if they were to bring to court the man who sold the drink. So I told the boys that prosecution was likely. They had not been in court before and were frightened at the prospect; and I was secretly concerned that a conditional discharge and a 'penny lecture' would not deter a second offence. So I said to them that when someone wronged someone else within the school, he took action to put things right; and in this case too there was something they could do rather than sit and worry. When they appeared in court, they were able to tell the magistrates how they had been down to the bus station on a Sunday morning and cleaned two buses which had been messed up on Saturday night; two of them had earned money to dry-clean the suede coat of a woman sitting next to the boy who was sick, and the third boy had printed a silk scarf for her. The magistrates were impressed, and told the boys that their own actions were more effective in dealing with the matter than any decision of the court's could have been. In this instance, it was not difficult to face both ways, because there was no fundamental clash of interests between the demands of the world and the needs of the boys; but the problem of how to turn the police's half-hearted decision to prosecute to the boys' advantage is an example of the problems which occur on the boundary.

The boundary has to enclose a space large enough for things (treatment, self-determination, play) to happen within it (Lampen 1978). Violence and apathy are two possible reactions to lack of space in this sense; and this may be seen as readily in a bad institution as in the Falls district of Belfast with its lack of opportunities for work, play and recreation. But this observation is not directly linked to the amount of programming or structuring within an establishment. A highly programmed day may enhance *or* restrict the individual's feeling of space to move, to grow and to be; expanses of open space and free time may be liberating *or* depressing and frightening. Many of our boys at Shotton Hall did not look forward to weekends, when we encouraged them to rely more on their own resources.

Similarly, the number of crossings of the boundary is not so important as the feeling that they are in safe hands. A setting specifically designed for psychotherapy, or a therapeutic community, provides space for things to happen by eliminating, or at least cutting down, the risk of intrusion by uncomprehending strangers. Settings offering family therapy, or work experience, will have many more comings and goings, but these will be carefully structured. The special problems of day-treatment centres are discussed by Foster (in Hinshelwood & Manning 1979). Leadership involves making decisions or eliciting group decisions on such matters as the arrival and departure of staff and inmates; the 'rights' of staff and the 'rights' or 'privileges' of clients in the matter of coming in and going out and inviting visitors; the degree of welcome for, or protection from, parents, social workers, police, officials, and people who service the institution. If such decisions are not made, and carried out, the boundary disintegrates. D W Winnicott (1965) once went so far as to suggest a treatment setting for disturbed children with a progression through five units. The last two would be concerned with reaching out across the boundary to normal family and school life; the admission unit would be comforting and protective. But in the second and third, the staff would have the task of 'covering naked souls', and outsiders would not be allowed to intrude. In most of our institutions all five units, with their diverse tasks and boundary needs, are rolled into one.

The internal boundaries

I heard some years ago of a children's home where the children, in general, spent the evening in a certain room. Near the fire was a small rug, and on the rug an armchair for the supervising staff member. The children were not allowed to use the chair, of course; but they were not even supposed to come on to the rug. This illustrates the contention of Goffman (1961) that establishments, starting with necessary aims, regulations and roles, 'add depth and colour to these arrangements'. How one speaks, what one does, where one goes, everything becomes determined by whether one has the role of staff or inmate. But to understand, let alone judge, the significance of that rug and armchair, one needs to ask: Who determined this arrangement? Do children ever come on to the rug? In what circumstances do they earn a reproof for doing so? and so on.

In a hierarchical establishment the head will set up the formal boundaries; in other situations these may be decided by the staff. In either case it remains a function of leadership to monitor them, and see that they contribute to the primary task, rather than work against it as the example given seems to do. A boundary may work against the task either by giving individual workers so little space that they cannot be creative or responsive – or so much space that anxiety kills these qualities in them.

At one time I was worried because boys were demanding to talk to houseparents late in the evening and I felt that many of the boys were manipulating staff in this. The Shotton Hall staff said they wanted to set the limits on when they could or could not see boys. I decided finally that they should continue to set this boundary, but I said that staff members who had boys in their rooms after ten o'clock were to tell me next day (even if it were their day off). The immediate result was that they refused most of the requests which they had previously allowed. But the more positive gain was that, a short time later, it became possible to discuss why these requests had been made and granted with a degree of frankness and insight not possible while the staff and I were competing over who should set this particular limit.

Even when the person in charge delineates the official boundaries within the establishment, the staff and clients will erect unauthorised ones of their own. This sometimes points to inadequate management of their anxieties. One of the most sensitive tasks of leadership is the removal of such frontiers when they seem to work against the primary task of the unit. In certain staff-management climates their removal may be impossible; and trades unions and professional associations can cross the external boundary and complicate the situation inside still further. Indeed, one of the strongest and most valid reasons for involving staff and to some extent clients in deciding on the 'official' internal boundaries, their purpose and effectiveness, is that it reduces the polarisation of staff and management and the re-interpretation of every question that comes up in terms of the polarity.

Apart from straightforward conflicts of interest, there will also be differences of opinion, heavily loaded with emotion, about how to act in particular situations. In my recollection, these were often over the question of whether to keep or exclude the most difficult boy at the time. I (usually with the support of one or two senior colleagues) accepted Winnicott's (1965) contention that there would always be one or two 'intolerable' children, and that to send them away was to fail not only them but the whole group. My fantasy about the boys was that they would see expulsion as our failure, and that other boys would react by trying to force us to expel them. My fantasy about the staff was that they were in the grip of a group panic, and that it would harm all of us if I were to 'give in' to their demands. Their fantasy about me was that I would always put the boys' needs higher than their needs, and the needs of the individual boy concerned above the needs of the group. Their fantasy about the boys was that the boys would see anything short of expulsion as weak leadership.

The Management of Anxiety

It can be argued that a certain amount of anxiety is an essential component in getting things done. Without it, many people are not punctual, tools do not get tidied away, communications are not improved nor situations clarified; workers do not feel the need to enlarge their understanding, and clients cannot be bothered to make progress.

But it can be argued with equal force that anxiety is a common disrupter of competent work, generating rigid and inappropriate procedures, paralysing the power of decision or forcing it to ill-considered action.

Since there is some truth in both viewpoints, and since people differ widely in the amount of anxiety they can use or even tolerate, the management of anxiety is a crucial task of leadership. A number of points can be made with some confidence.

(i)   *'Unnecessary' anxieties should be eliminated by the person in charge.* By 'unnecessary' I mean anxieties which can only hinder the establishment in carrying out its tasks. Thus, in most establishments, uncertainty about who is to cook lunch would be wholly unjustifiable. At Finchden Manor, however, it was justified because it was part of a conscious treatment strategy, and hence 'necessary'. Anxieties originating outside the boundary are very often anti-task. If leadership cannot protect the staff from them (as in the case of threatened closure) it is axiomatic that the work will suffer.

(ii)   *When necessary or inevitable anxieties arise, leadership must decide whether to refer them for solution inside or outside the boundary.*

(iii)   *When anxiety is to be dealt with inside the boundary, leadership must be clear about the alternative strategies.* Broadly speaking, the choice is likely to be between strengthening some aspect of the defensive structure (rules, routines, punishments) or working on some aspect of group or individual psycho-dynamics. The decision, however it is reached, must take account of the goals of the establishment as well as the level of anxiety being felt.

(iv)   *Leadership may sometimes tolerate (or even generate) a certain amount of anxiety to challenge staff defences.*

(v)   *Situations involving great anxiety should be examined together by all the professional workers involved in them when the crisis is over.* Sometimes this evokes so much renewed anxiety that it is tempting not to do so.

The uncertainty involved in the therapeutic situation can arouse great anxiety, but this uncertainty defines the space within which helper and helped can create something positive (Winnicott 1974). Unnecessary and overwhelming anxieties need to be dissipated to free the resources of the worker (nurse, houseparent, social therapist, educator, doctor) to cope with this creative uncertainty.

The Nurture of Junior Staff

Some settings have a static task, such as the supervision of custodial sentences; but almost all settings for adolescents envisage positive change during their stay in the institution, and so have a dynamic aspect. The static task can largely be performed by routine procedures; but even here, leadership's task of building up staff morale is important. In the dynamic setting, much less is covered by routines, since the patient's personal development largely occurs within the area of uncertainty already mentioned. The use of this 'open space' need not be frightening; it can lead to increased staff commitment, skill and satisfaction. But this will depend on how well the workers are cared for. Even in behaviour modification regimes, which are committed to set procedures, experienced practitioners draw attention to the crucial importance of creative imagination and staff training and support (Brown 1979; Burland 1979).

Leadership has the following responsibilities towards new and junior staff:

(i)   *Training in specific procedures and regulations.*

(ii) *Establishment of two-way trust.* The member of staff needs to believe in the leadership's competence and concern; the leader(s) need confidence in the worker's strength and sensitivity. Often trust is not fully established until after some shared difficult experiences.

(iii) *Giving the worker scope and challenge.* Observation and intuition should suggest where the worker can be given space to improvise and experiment, and where clear directives are needed either to protect the worker (where he or she is felt to be at risk) or to bring out latent abilities.

(iv) *Giving support.* This includes dispassionate analysis of events, and help in achieving self-understanding; encouragement, criticisms, prohibitions, detailed instructions, at times comfort; also preparation for enlarging the worker's 'space'.

(v)   *Providing a model.* In acting in these ways towards the worker, leadership is providing a model of how the worker should care for, guide and challenge the client. The worker is likely to imitate leadership's direct relations with the clients: how concern is expressed, problems and confrontations are negotiated, and authority is used.

(vi) *Understanding a staff member's development.* This means a degree of empathy with the alternation of positive and depressed feelings about the demands of the work, with ideals and resistances. It includes the ability to accept the worker's idealisation of the leader, or anger, without feeling flattered or threatened.

On one occasion at Shotton Hall, a housemother came to say that a boy had threatened to hit her with a piece of metal. She had given this boy, whose behaviour was eccentric but not usually aggressive, a number of individual play sessions, and she and I had felt there was the beginning of trust between them. On this occasion she had reminded him that it was his bath-night, and had asked him to give her his trousers afterwards which were long overdue for the laundry. His reluctance to change his clothes regularly had been noticed by other staff, and she had felt she had a good chance of persuading him. His reaction had moved from gruff refusal to signs of distress, which were quickly covered up; he then seized the metal and threatened to hit her if she did not go away. She did not feel that he wanted to make an attack.

My reaction was quite specific to what I knew of this worker from regular weekly supervision sessions and seeing her with boys, and from my hunch about the boy. When I felt sure she was not really frightened, but puzzled and alarmed by the incident, and guilty about walking out on it, I suggested there was something very painful for him in all this – so painful that he was prepared to inflict the pain on someone he liked, if only he could drive it away from himself. How would she feel about going straight back to him, not to press the matter of the trousers, but to say she felt his pain, and could he find a way to share it with her by talking instead of by hitting? She did so, and a long conversation that evening was followed by many more. A long time afterwards, the boy told me how her return and her challenge 'felt like a bucket of water in the face. It's as if I was sleep-walking up to then'.

Models of Leadership

A treatment setting is dependent on the world around it to survive, at the levels of policy, referrals, and basic material needs. Yet its members are being encouraged to work through 'crazy' patterns of behaviour. These two things are only compatible given firm, understanding, incorruptible and skilful leadership. Poor leadership can be identified by a number of linked symptoms: poor boundary definition and maintenance; pervasive uncertainty about the ethos or its application to actual practice; excessive anxiety; staff and clients not feeling cared for and challenged. Such faults are not the prerogative of any profession, and it is clear that the authority conferred by professional expertise does not in itself provide the certainty of good leadership. I believe, too, that the acceptibility of a leader to a multi-disciplinary team will ultimately depend on the traits described in this chapter, rather than on professional background, although that will probably be the most important factor in establishing and justifying the ethos of the establishment. Perhaps good leaders, like good therapists, are born as much as made; but I think that suitable people could be greatly helped by being trained to function in the ways that I have described.

After all this discussion, can we establish the advantages and disadvantages of different models of leadership? There are four models which are relevant.

(i)   The single authority-figure at the apex of a hierarchical delegating pyramid. This traditional British and American pattern assumes that wisdom resides with the senior person, by virtue of experience and authority. It provides the leader with strong support. Some attempts at checks and safeguards (and lip-service to the concept of democracy) are generally provided in the form of an overseeing committee. But pity the committee – unable to watch the processes under discussion – which has to decide whether, in a particular instance, wisdom was on the side of the head or a staff group united against him. The film *The Caine Mutiny* (based on a novel by Hermann Wouk) gave a fascinating illustration of this dilemma, and showed how the scales of justice will tend to tip towards legitimate authority.

The single leader has to bear the 'powerlessness' of all the other staff on his shoulders without becoming tyrannous, manipulated or indecisive. The pressures of what people project on to him or her are formidable; personal support, most needed by this type of leadership, is often not provided.

(ii)   An individual head who takes a high degree of responsibility with regard to the outside boundary, but allows for autonomy and initiative internally, relating to staff members (individually and as professional groupings) as a consultant with a residual authority to fall back on. This may also include a measure of client participation (Lampen 1978). This system seems to me to meet most of the criteria of this chapter, but exposes the leader to considerable pressures, since her or his particular blend of control and permissiveness is unlikely to suit everyone in the establishment. Typically, staff may feel that they need more latitude, the clients less; and it is not uncommon for contradictory demands to come from a single ambivalent source. This style of leadership allows the leader to benefit from the expertise of the different professional disciplines on the staff team, but may require a lot of time and tact in monitoring the boundaries between them (which the first model of leadership decides by dictatorial *fiat*).

(iii) A system in which the most senior members of the professional disciplines involved form a managing committee. This would avoid the problems inherent in having a single leader; it might well be used more widely, if it were not that the key factor of the leaders' interpersonal relationship is so unpredictable. It has been said that behind every form of government there lies an oligarchy; this system would have the advantage of bringing it into the open, and assuring junior staff that their professional viewpoint was fully represented in policy. The fact that this is theoretically possible, but so seldom found in practice, highlights the problems which do arise in single-leadership settings which have a multiple task of care, treatment and education.

(iv)   A truly democratic staff group (which may or may not also have a component of client participation). We know still less about this model than the preceding one, so any conclusions must be very tentative. The most obvious objection is that the institution exists to do a skilled task, which needs experienced management, and the relevant techniques are not an appropriate matter to subject to majority vote. The most obvious advantage, the sense of partnership in all staff, can be obtained in other ways. A further objection is that the tasks of leadership, particularly the maintenance of the internal and external boundaries, would take up so much of the time available for debate and decision making, and would be so subject to the intermittent change characteristic of democratic processes, that the efficiency and security of the establishment would suffer. But these points are speculative; and it would be most valuable to have some accounts of fully democratic leadership, carefully described and evaluated. There are some suggestive and encouraging studies from other fields in Gibson (1979).

The model of leadership is clearly crucial to the process of decision-making; and the four described might be expected to provide a spectrum from maximum consistency and continuity through to maximum adaptability. But I doubt whether this would be found true in practice. Decision-making is not one single process; and it is different in relation to long-term aims, choice of the treatment methods, and here-and-now decisions. Long-term goals are often set by external authority; but leadership is responsible for assessing whether they are practical and being achieved. It is also concerned with the relationship of primary to secondary goals, as Balburnie (1966) points out. For instance, what is the status of education within a psychiatric unit, or psychotherapy in a special school? Decisions in this area should not be too easy to change, or the whole enterprise will feel as though it had shifting foundations.

The choice of the means of treatment involves more complex questions. Each strategy has to be considered from at least five viewpoints:

(i)   *Is it morally right?* We can never guarantee results; but we are responsible for the means we implement. Therefore we can never justify them solely in terms of the goal aimed at.

(ii) *Is it compatible with the other strategies being used?*

(iii) *Is it effective?* The type of leadership will influence the question of who evaluates results and how they do so.

(iv) *What effect does it have on the systems and subsystems of communication?* Systems theory has shown how the style of communication between leader and staff, for example, will be mirrored in staff-inmate exchanges. Certain strategies, appropriate to their aims, will fail if they work against the grain of the prevailing pattern of decision-making and communication.

(v)   *Is it sufficiently flexible?* If the primary task is static, as in a local prison, procedures which can be adapted to small differences in situation will tend to cause anxiety and resentment in staff and inmates. In education, physical and psychiatric medicine, the consumer is generally expected to develop from dependence to independence; procedures which are rigid may fail to meet his or her changing needs.

Decision-making in the immediate situation forms a great deal of the work of leadership. But we should not forget that the majority of the here-and-now decisions are being made by staff without reference to higher authority. The cumulative effect of these decisions is subtly reshaping the treatment methods and even the long-term aims all the time. Leadership may try to control this by detailed directives, but I believe that sympathetic supervision with plenty of dialogue is more effective. Staff training sessions should include help in handling immediate situations effectively without prejudicing long-term goals, along the lines suggested by Redl & Wineman (1952).

Conclusion

I do not believe that any model of leadership is uniquely suited to any particular set of goals. Contrary to stereotyped expectations, there are collective leaderships which are rigid and defensive, and autocrats who are flexible, sensitive, and encouragers of initiative. The relationship between the human 'establishment', the tasks of the institution, the strategies adopted, and the external environment, is a complex and pervasive one which cannot be reduced to a formula. But that is no excuse for lack of self-awareness in this vital area. For while there is no one 'right' solution, it is also true that unscrutinised systems are often working against the task in blatant as well as subtle ways.

References and Further Reading

Balburnie R (1966) *Residential Work with Children*. Oxford: Pergamon Press
Brown P J (1979) A theoretical and practical account of behaviour modification. *A WMC Journal*, **7**(2)
Burland J R (1979) Behaviour modification in a residential school for junior maladjusted boys: an overview. *A WMC Journal*, **7**(2)
Davies Jones H (1970) *Leadership in Residential Child Care*. London: National Children's Home
Gibson T (1979) *People Power*. Harmondsworth: Penguin
Goffman E (1961) *Asylums* New York: Doubleday; Harmondsworth: Penguin (1968)
Greenleaf R K (1977) *Servant Leadership*. New York: Paulist Press
Hinshelwood R D & Manning N (1979) *Therapeutic Communities: Reflections and Progress*. London: Routledge & Kegan Paul
Jones M (1976) *The Maturation of the Therapeutic Community*. New York: Human Sciences Press
Lampen J C (1978) Drest in a little brief authority. *Journal of Adolescence*, **1**(2)
Redl F, Wineman D (1952) *Controls from Within*. New York: Free Press
Rice A K (1965) *The Enterprise and its Environment*. London: Tavistock Press
Rice A K (1965) *Learning for Leadership*. London: Tavistock Press
Winnicott D W (1965) *The Maturational Process and the Facilitating Environment*. London: Hogarth Press
Winnicott D W (1974) *Playing and Reality*. Harmondsworth: Penguin

The Adolescent Unit
Edited by Derek Steinberg
© 1986 D. Steinberg

19 Multidisciplinary Teamwork: Help or Hindrance?

William Ll Parry-Jones

I entered my present work with adolescents from general rather than child psychiatry. Such a step would be less likely today, but I believe that adolescent psychiatrists need to have a thorough and continuing familiarity with the management of adult patients, because this promotes a more realistic understanding of the natural history and prognosis of adolescent disorders. I am actively interested in the planning and delivery of psychiatric services for adolescents which are both as comprehensive as possible and cost-effective, and in the provision of short-term, eclectic treatment. My long-standing involvement in research into the history of psychiatry has encouraged me to adopt, at all times, a critical, even sceptical approach towards psychiatric practice, especially currently fashionable treatments and patterns of care.

———◆———

Most people are likely to regard the multidisciplinary team as one of the central features of day-to-day practice in the delivery of services for disturbed adolescents. Its *raison d'être* may seem self-evident, but it is rarely challenged or dissected analytically. In fact, it has acquired the trappings of a 'sacred cow', with more attention being focused on making it work than on its meaning and justification. The history of psychiatry makes abundantly clear the pitfall of unquestioning acceptance of any currently fashionable approaches and organisational models of care. It follows that the multidisciplinary team should not be sacrosanct and exempt from critical scrutiny. Instead, questions need to be asked openly about whether it is the most efficient way of deploying scarce manpower, how effective it is in promoting the highest standards of patient care and to what extent it serves to advance the practice and knowledge of adolescent psychiatry. In this chapter, some aspects of multidisciplinary teamwork in adolescent psychiatry are probed. It is a wide and complex field and no attempt is made to cover it comprehensively.

Historical Background

Collaboration between doctors and nursing attendants became an established feature of the asylum system in the eighteenth century, although medical authority was unchallenged and the status of psychiatric nurses remained low until comparatively recent decades. In the 1920s, the growth of the Child Guidance Movement was associated closely with the emergence of a new form of interdisciplinary practice involving psychiatrists, psychologists and social workers. This particular pattern of collaboration has continued to shape the organisation of services for disturbed children and adolescents, with the gradual addition of other professional workers, such as child psychotherapists. In the 1950s and 1960s, the exciting concept of the 'therapeutic community' swept through mental hospitals, disrupting the time-honoured equilibrium of bureaucratic organisation and blurring the roles of staff set in profession-centred ways of working. At the same time, rapid development began to take place in the separate professional identities of the various non-medical disciplines involved in the care of psychiatric patients, leading to enlarged and reinforced hierarchic organisations and heightened self-concern about professional autonomy. The scene was set for rivalry, power struggles and conflict about leadership and the division of labour between doctors, nurses, psychologists, social workers and other professional staff. Working together in the day-to-day care of patients, however, staff had to find new formulae for harmonious coexistence and therapeutic efficacy. The notion of the multidisciplinary 'team' emerged as a solution – an expedient way of concealing, or at best partially resolving, inter-professional tensions. It was in this climate, in the late 1960s, that adolescent psychiatry was established, mainly in geographically scattered regional units. Not surprisingly, in such a new field, the operational policies of these early units developed along diverse, experimental lines and were influenced by the prevailing philosophy of the therapeutic community and a mood of 'anti-psychiatry'. Doubts about whether 'illness' or 'social distress' were the crucial issues in disorder and treatment were reinforced by the increasing input of non-medical disciplines. From the outset, the multidisciplinary team was an accepted part of services. Despite its merits, this policy has been slow to mature, hamstrung by issues concerned with professional status and confused by the mirage of the 'ideal' team, free from internal group conflicts.

'Modus Operandi' and Pros and Cons of Multidisciplinary Teams

The term multidisciplinary team tends to be used loosely, usually with the implication that it refers to one distinct entity. But, in fact, it can mean very different things to different disciplines and probably this confusion has been one of the factors contributing to all the problems attributed to teamwork. A useful starting point in the search for clarification and definition is provided by two Working Papers of the Brunel Institute of Organisation and Social Studies (BIOSS) concerned, respectively, with the organisation of Child Guidance and allied work (1976) and with the nature and function of multidisciplinary work in services for the mentally ill (Rowbottom and Hey, 1978). In both Papers, a clear distinction is drawn between 'teams' and 'networks'. The following definition of a team is proposed (BIOSS 1976): 'A situation where practitioners work together who: (a) are personally known to each other; (b) are mutually acceptable as co-members; (c) intend to work together for an indefinite period; (d) work face-to-face with each other in greater or smaller numbers, and frequently face-to-face as a whole group. Team membership implies: (a) the right of pre-existing members, other than those in clearly subordinate positions . . . to veto the appointment or attachment of new members; (b) the right to be included in all general team discussions; (c) the duty to abide by established norms and procedures of interaction'. By contrast (Rowbottom & Hey, 1978) a feature of working in networks is that 'Small groups or "teams" may meet for particular tasks or particular occasions, but there exists no one permanent and definite face-to-face group . . . face-to-face work may be sporadic. Individuals may come and go (for example according to shift-work and duty-systems) . . . the staff associated with some particular ward in a hospital – perhaps numbering several dozen, with individuals continually coming and going – are often better thought of as members of a large network though frequently described as a team.' A central issue is made, in the second Working Paper, of the fact that there is no single, unambiguous pattern of teamwork and the variables that can determine different patterns of teamwork are explored. These include the ways in which authority and responsibility are are explored. These include the ways in which authority and responsibility are distributed, the experience and expectations of the participants and the extent to which they operate at the same level, and the particular conceptual framework about psychiatric disorder that is adopted.

A number of reports approach multidisciplinary work from the viewpoint of particular disciplines. For example, in a report on *The Role of Psychologists in the Health Service* (DHSS 1977) an attempt was made to reconcile, within multi-disciplinary teamwork, the possible independent professional status of clinical psychologists with the continuing medical responsibility of psychiatrists. The interpretation of teamwork proposed was that it 'implies the mutual recognition, by the members of the different professions concerned, of a shared responsibility for patient care. This does not . . . mean that every decision affecting a patient will necessarily be a team decision. Each profession has its own sphere of competence and its members are responsible for their decisions within that sphere. They are also individually responsible for recognising the limits of their own competence and enlisting the involvement of their colleagues when this becomes necessary. The decisions which involve the team as a whole are those concerning the patient's care as a whole which involve a choice between different forms of professional intervention.'

The important delineation between team-functioning at the clinical level and that at management and administrative levels was made by the Royal College of Psychiatrists (1977). This is a useful distinction because of the particular difficulties in establishing an agreed approach towards teamwork in the care of individual patients, partly because of contention about the nature of medical responsibility.

Another clear point made by the Royal College of Psychiatrists is that 'multi-disciplinary team functioning should be seen as an option, not as a rigid pattern, and there should be discretion at ward level.'

Whilst multidisciplinary work covers a wide range of practices, some common problems can be identified. The main difficulties have arisen in relation to questions about the parity and division of authority amongst the participants. Such problems have occurred particularly clearly in traditionally-structured Child Guidance Services and have been described by the Inter-disciplinary Standing Committee (1981) and in a BIOSS Working Paper (1976). The issue of leadership arises readily in the work-setting of a permanent or semipermanent team structure made up of experienced professionals. The authority exercised by the consultant psychiatrist is a particularly sensitive issue because in the treatment of individual patients, the legal, ethical, diagnostic and prescriptive responsibilities of doctors cannot be delegated to the multidisciplinary team. A number of basic assumptions about how teams should be organised, irrespective of the service required, may be responsible for intra-group tension and ill-feeling. Perhaps the most common are that all team members should be 'equal', that all decisions have to be mediated through the team and that no single member should be able to veto team decisions. It is clear that, whilst these features may be workable in certain teams, in other situations they may be simply impracticable.

One of the characteristic features of work in the mental health field is that it is hard to differentiate clearly between the appropriate professional contributions of staff. This problem is accentuated if the prevailing theoretical model is more concerned with social dysfunction than with 'illness'. Whilst profession-centred role responsibilities may become difficult to define, however, the scope for what may be called 'unidisciplinary' practice increases. Substantial involvement in such areas offers one way of resolving inter-professional tensions. This solution is shown particularly clearly in the adoption of the therapeutic community or family therapy approaches as the principal patterns of care. One of the key recommendations of the Inter-disciplinary Standing Committee was that the understanding and management of rivalries and conflicts within the team should be one of the skills required by all the disciplines concerned. This is a time-consuming process because issues concerned with authority relationships between interacting professionals, and especially those involving the prescribing authority, are highly complex. It raises the question of whether conflict has to be accepted as an inevitable feature, and, if so, whether the potential benefits of teamwork outweigh its inherent disadvantages.

Day-to-day practice in adolescent psychiatry, however, makes it clear that combined professional work is crucial. Adolescent disturbance covers a wide spectrum of disorder, generating diverse needs and demanding a variety of services. No single professional group, service or agency has the capacity to manage all aspects of all cases, and it is good practice to bring to bear on problems every available specialist resource and skill. Since there is no single, all-purpose model of multidisciplinary work, the organisation of the ways in which professional people work together needs to be very carefully planned to match the services required. The following account of combined professional work in an adolescent unit provides an illustration of how this has been accomplished in one centre.

Multidisciplinary Work at Highfield, the Oxford Regional Psychiatric Adolescent Unit

Highfield receives some 400 referrals annually, from a total population of 2.5 million. All referrals are routed through medical sources to the two consultant psychiatrists, who maintain close contact with general practitioners. In this account, attention will be focused chiefly on interdisciplinary work in the inpatient unit.

This 16-bedded unit is characterised by an emphasis on short stay, on the intake of patients within a wide diagnostic range and on the acceptance of emergency admissions. The general orientation is based on the clinical psychiatric model and there is an eclectic approach to treatment, always involving close contact with parents. The unit is not run as a therapeutic community, but instead, emphasis is placed on the intensive assessment and treatment of individual adolescents and their families. In recent years, there have been up to 100 admissions annually, with an average length of stay of 5–7 weeks. The staff comprises four psychiatrists (two consultants), 17 nurses (one full-time senior nurse), three psychologists (two senior posts), two teachers, one social work co-ordinator, one senior occupational therapist, two secretaries and two domestic staff. In addition, there are always several supernumerary staff on training placements. The responsibility of the two consultant psychiatrists for providing and developing services and their independent practitioner status distinguishes them from fully-trained practitioners in other disciplines, such as the senior clinical psychologists, the senior nurse and the senior occupational therapist, who do not operate at consultant level, and also from trainees and students.

Interdisciplinary collaboration takes different forms according to the specific tasks being undertaken and falls into three broad groups.

1 Management and administration

The operational policy has undergone progressive change over the last fifteen years, being clarified and developed by successive generations of staff. One consultant psychiatrist is designated in administrative charge of the unit. This responsibility carries very little managerial power, since apart from trainee psychiatrists, all the other staff are part of extended hierarchies within their own professions. Nevertheless, there is considerable scope for leadership in relation to the co-ordination of activities and the functional evolution of the unit, whilst acknowledging fully the managerial responsibilities of the other senior professional staff. The consultant in administrative charge chairs the monthly Management Group, attended by the senior members of all the disciplines. This core, multidisciplinary group remains relatively unchanged for long periods, and is concerned with the overall management of the unit, the continuing review of its work, and with forward planning.

In addition, there are weekly Staff Policy Meetings, chaired rotationally by members of each discipline, at which all matters concerning the daily functioning of the unit are discussed and through which all proposals for policy change are routed. These meetings are conducted formally, with a planned agenda and typed minutes. Sub-committees and working-parties are formed regularly to undertake specific tasks and projects such as redrafting policy documents, and these provide additional opportunities for the dispersal of leadership functions.

2 Clinical work

Highfield is an NHS unit, whose work is a 'mental health-orientated' activity and the two consultant psychiatrists carry the ultimate or prime responsibility for the care of the patients referred to them. Consequently, they have general leadership responsibilities for the staff working on specific cases. It is the general policy of the unit to delineate, as clearly as possible, the central role responsibilities of all staff, to provide structure and consistency and to make explicit their distinctive skills and knowledge. The attempt made by Rowbottom and Hey (1978) to describe the 'distinctive competences' of various professional groups is a useful starting point for clarification. For example, social workers have 'knowledge of family and community social systems, and of a wide range of agencies, services and social provisions; special skills in helping people to gain a better relationship within their normal social environment.' These tend to be rather non-specific 'competences' and the social work co-ordinator's role at Highfield includes special responsibility for chairing the weekly Family Work Review Meeting, for allocating family workers, and for organising family therapy training. Within this organisational framework, multidisciplinary collaboration operates in three ways.

(i) *Individual case teams.* These are an important part of the day-to-day clinical practice of the unit. They comprise the nurse allocated to the patient, the family worker(s), a psychiatrist and any other member of staff involved in the case for a particular reason, for example, a teacher or occupational therapist. Case teams are expected to plan, co-ordinate and carry out the main part of the assessment and treatment of individual patients and their families. Treatment programmes and progress are reviewed at the weekly Ward Round, chaired by the consultant psychiatrists. It is the custom for the family worker, usually a very experienced member of staff, to be responsible for convening meetings. Disagreement about leadership is rare, although sometimes, there is a failure to nominate a convenor in an appropriately clear way.

(ii) *Open, multidisciplinary clinical meetings.* All staff with duties on the inpatient unit are expected to attend a number of daily and weekly meetings concerning all inpatients, including the Ward Round and the Family Work Review Meeting. These provide an opportunity for staff at all levels to make a contribution to the clinical work, irrespective of discipline or status, and to the common clinical tasks of getting patients better. They create invaluable occasions for pooling information, generating new ideas, and facilitating communication.

(iii) *Collaboration in overlap areas of unidisciplinary work.* Some therapeutic skills employed in psychiatry are not the prerogative of any single profession, for example certain forms of individual counselling and psychotherapy, family therapy, social skills training and the leadership of small groups. All of these are important components of treatment at Highfield and participation is more dependent on personal qualities, experience and training than on professional labels. The ideal of everyone contributing according to their talents can be attained most closely in such work and it enables individuals from various disciplines to make leadership contributions, without the conflict and frustrations that indiscriminate role-blurring can generate. The family worker(s) in case teams, therefore, can be drawn from any professional group, other than the teachers, whose agreed commitment excludes this work and, in addition, small group leaders have been selected in this way.

3 In-service training

Each professional group is responsible for the specific instruction and supervision of its trainees, but this leaves considerable scope for interdisciplinary training and supervision groups, the latter an opportunity to discuss personal and professional matters in a case-related way. It is the policy, however, not to have sensitivity groups concerned with staff interaction. In part, this is because of the unhelpful levels of anxiety about identity and the insecurity that may be generated, and also because 'opening up and communicating' can take the place, insidiously, of work function.

The size of the total staff group at Highfield, its constantly changing nature and the inherent differences in status and levels of work, mean that it should not be regarded as a multidisciplinary 'team' but as a 'network', within which various collaborative activities can occur. It is only in the case teams that clinical teamwork is practised in anything approaching a pure form, and even then on a temporary case-related basis. This overall structure, utilising short-term work groups, reduces fears of interdisciplinary conflict by the knowledge that alternative assignments are always available. Whilst input, at all levels, from various disciplines is valued highly, the process of 'teamwork' as such is not an over-riding preoccupation. There is shared appreciation of professional skills, knowledge and allegiances. In this respect, the author has always respected the way in which the constraints imposed by medical responsibility and confidentiality have been acknowledged and accepted by colleagues. The dual influence on staff of both the Highfield 'team' and of separate professional and management hierarchies, with the consequent risks of divided loyalties, is recognised. Both intra- and interdisciplinary meetings, therefore, are part of the established practice.

Conclusion

There is no single pattern of teamwork that is universally applicable or desirable – there are no standard rules. Indeed, the indiscriminate use of the term multi-disciplinary team serves to conceal and depreciate the potential scope of inter-professional collaboration.

Traditional bureaucratic and 'egalitarian' organisational structures both have disadvantages. Maintaining a compromise between these two models, nevertheless, is like walking the proverbial tightrope. The brief description of the forms of combined professional work undertaken at Highfield, illustrates the variety of ways in which 'teams' may operate, usually on a temporary basis, within a multidisciplinary 'network'. This model obviates some of the problems that arise in 'permanent' teamwork.

Practical choices have to be made about the way staff collaborate in relation to particular tasks. These have to take into consideration, in an open and realistic way, differences in the status and levels of competence of the staff and the fact that they are not necessarily collaborating as equals. Each individual, from different disciplines, has to find his or her own role. This process is determined by the interaction of personality, professional training, formal role structures as well as opportunities for spontaneous contribution and planned role-blurring. Experience of the success of this flexible model leads the author to the conclusion that a rigid, idealised view of long-lasting multidisciplinary team functioning, with all the well-rehearsed arguments about authority relationships based on the ethos of equality, is outmoded. It is not in the best interests of high quality patient care; it impedes the development of individual professions and the advancement of adolescent psychiatry as a whole. All the recommendations that have been made for improving the quality of teamwork will have little effect unless there is full acceptance of the need for diversity and flexibility in combined professional work.

References and Further Reading

Brunel Institute of Organisation and Social Studies (BIOSS) (1976) *Working Paper H/S1. Future Organisation in Child Guidance and Allied Work.* London: Brunel University

Department of Health and Social Security (1977) *The Role of Psychologists in the Health Services* (Trethowan). London: HMSO

Inter-disciplinary Standing Committee (1981) *Multi-disciplinary Work in Child Guidance.* Child Guidance Trust

Royal College of Psychiatrists (1977) The responsibilities of consultants in psychiatry within the National Health Service. *Bulletin of the Royal College of Psychiatrists*, September, 4–7

Royal College of Psychiatrists (1978) The role, responsibilities and work of the child and adolescent psychiatrist. *Bulletin of the Royal College of Psychiatrists*, July, 127–131

Rowbottom R & Hey A (1978) *Organisation of Services for the Mentally Ill – A Working Paper.* London: Brunel Institute of Organisation and Social Studies (BIOSS)

The Adolescent Unit
Edited by Derek Steinberg
© 1986 D. Steinberg

20 Trainees in the Multidisciplinary Team: A Worm's Eye View

Adrian Angold

> *'Jack Barrett went to Quetta*
> *Because they told him to'*
> Kipling

Having been brought up and educated in London and the Home Counties, I received my medical training at the London Hospital Medical College. During this time I developed an interest in psychology and gained an intercalated BSc in that subject. Following house jobs in London, I joined the SHO/Registrar training rotation at the Bethlem Royal and Maudsley Hospitals. After eighteen months in adult psychiatric posts, I decided to pursue a career in child psychiatry during a child guidance placement. This was followed by six months as registrar in the Adolescent Unit at Bethlem. I have research interests in a number of areas but particularly in depression in childhood.

———◆———

Much of this book is written by people with a more or less long-term commitment to a particular multidisciplinary team. However, this team has as one of its major functions the training of transient members of various disciplines in placements of varying duration. My own experience of it was on a six-month placement as a psychiatric registrar in a training rotation. Nevertheless the discussion which follows is relevant to other professionals passing through a multidisciplinary unit as part of higher specialist training, for example, as social workers, nurses or clinical psychologists.

Trainees Need Teams

Work with disturbed children and their families is complex and demanding and the skills required are diverse and distributed among the members of various disciplines. As the 1977 report of the WHO Expert Committee on Child Mental Health and Psychosocial Development states, 'The mental health of children is inextricably linked with their psychosocial development, so that all those concerned with the growth and development of children and with the process of socialisation and education can contribute to the promotion of child mental health. Services should therefore be provided jointly by health workers, teachers, social workers and others.

These workers need to have close communication in their daily work and divide among themselves responsibilities for different tasks.' Furthermore, authority in relation to child care may be placed in the hands of a variety of professionals, for instance, teachers in the case of most children or social workers when children are in the care of a local authority. The trainee in any of these areas requires contact with members of a range of other disciplines. The best way of doing this is, surely, to work closely in a clinical setting with these other professionals.

Multidisciplinary teams are by no means a new phenomenon (Ackerly 1947), and it is perhaps a measure of the need for experience and training in their operation that it still remains a difficult task to establish and run such a team successfully. Of course, the necessary processes of adaptation may sometimes be difficult to endure and some will find that teamwork threatens their sense of professional competence and identity, and be unable to use the resources of the team to their advantage. Some team members may also have an interest, conspicuous or otherwise, in not helping to develop the skills of trainees of other disciplines, or even in undermining them. This is not the place to list all the pathologies of teams, but consideration of the points made in this chapter may help each trainee to develop his own nosology and formulate strategies for surviving on multidisciplinary battlefields.

An elegant statement of the conflicts and advantages to be found in working with others has been provided by Henry Maudsley in a discussion of the social development of the human species (Maudsley 1902). 'Two persons meeting in frequent intercourse soon find that they cannot enjoy a state of perfect liberty, that they must needs bear and forbear, and, secondly, that by living in social union each gains largely in power and comfort'. Support for this view in relation to junior medical staff in a therapeutic community for adolescents has recently been provided by Wells (1984) whose survey revealed considerable satisfaction with the opportunities for professional and personal growth afforded by such a setting.

Teams Need Trainees

It is a common complaint of multidisciplinary teams that trainees stay too short a time, and that the task of integrating them into the team is exhausting and redirects team resources away from their clients. It has been argued, indeed, that stability of personnel is a *sine qua non* for effective teamwork (Bettelheim 1974; Wilson 1979). Such a view carries the corollary that trainees are inimical to teamwork, since they are not permanently committed to the team.

There can be no doubt that providing a good training experience is very demanding and that certain old issues recur with every new trainee. Staff groups constantly repeat the cycle of greeting and getting used to new members, making decisions about how to use them and be used by them, and then saying goodbye. This roundabout is often regretted. No doubt some trainees will be idle or incompetent too, or just plain unpleasant to work with. However, trainees can also confer very considerable benefits on otherwise stable teams. At the most obvious level, they may do a lot of work, thereby increasing the productivity of the team. Moreover, they may be given some of the more basic and tedious work (such as writing up case histories), on the perhaps spurious grounds that they need this experience. There is also a certain kudos which attaches to having trainees, and being able to claim a significant training function may help a team to maintain its levels of staffing and finance. Furthermore, any discipline with a trainee thereby increases its level of representation in the team, which may be advantageous in team politics.

Many people of course actually enjoy providing teaching and supervision and would miss trainees if they were to disappear. And at least some trainees will be interesting, stimulating people with many useful ideas of their own to offer. By changing the constellation of professional relationships and stirring the interdisciplinary pudding, either by accident or intent, trainees may help to prevent stagnation in teams where permanent members stay for a long time.

Other, more subtle, advantages exist. In a sense, as mentioned above, the new trainee represents a threat to the team. Perhaps he will be no good, perhaps he will offend members of other disciplines! But his advent provides the team with a task about which all are likely to agree; he must be initiated into the ways of the team and encouraged to act accordingly throughout his stay. He may be important therefore in cementing the team together with a sort of Dunkirk spirit in the face of his potential dangerousness.

Where trainees of one discipline are clearly seen as subordinate to the established team members of the other disciplines they may thereby help to raise the general level of self-esteem and defuse interdisciplinary jealousies. At best, such conflicts may be sublimated into a helpful and protective attitude towards juniors of another discipline, though there is also scope for the trainee to be used as a scapegoat and vehicle for the expression of interdisciplinary rivalries. Should this last danger become a reality, or better still to anticipate it, the permanent staff should probably set up some forum (a 'senior staff' or 'core staff' group perhaps) to allow them to work out their differences among themselves (see Chapter 21). Such a move carries the drawback of producing in the trainee something of a feeling of alienation from the team, and the writer has had the uncomfortable experience of being one of three trainees excluded from a meeting of 'core staff' discussing a particular problem which had training implications. It should also be borne in mind that such a move will reduce his experience of certain important conflicts and management tasks; but overall this price is probably worth paying, if it helps the team to provide integrated and coherent training and support and, in general, set a good example.

The Experience

Having outlined briefly why the team and the trainee need each other, let us consider in more detail what each can bring to, and expect of, the other.

The Trainee's experience

People undergoing higher specialist training are expected to have a certain general level of expertise within their discipline and informed opinions about patients or clients. They may also belong to a professional organisation or union. Thus, the psychiatric registrar is expected to be able to perform a competent physical examination, unsupervised, and present an opinion on the patient's physical health. He is considered sufficiently responsible for his decisions and actions to be required by law to be insured with one of the medical defence societies. Yet he cannot function entirely as an independent practitioner and must submit to supervision by his seniors (senior registrars and consultants). Furthermore, his training placement may have involved little choice on his part and even less on the part of most of the rest of the team; nor could he expect necessarily to become a permanent member of the team he joins. Moreover, the trainee may start his placement with little idea of the work involved and even less of staff relationships in the team. He needs to learn about both very quickly. The first impression he makes is important and often resistant to change, while in a few short months his supervisor will be writing reports or references which will affect his future career. He may also find that, as a member of his particular profession, certain special skills may be attributed to him which he may not feel he actually possesses.

If he has already had experience of well-functioning multidisciplinary teams, the trainee will know roughly what to expect and may have discovered certain key concepts of multidisciplinary work (like the difference between supervision and consultation). His demonstration of this knowledge will help everyone to relax a little and be a useful step towards his being perceived positively by the team. He might also be used to observing who has power in relation to what and then modifying his behaviour accordingly. This often means keeping out of matters which belong principally to another discipline (or, at least, are felt to do so) until some right to become involved in them has been established. For instance, where social workers are the principal family work practitioners in the team, the doctor should not assume that his own views, experience or training in this field immediately qualify him to take a lead in discussion. On the other hand, he will be expected to demonstrate immediate competence in areas assigned by the team to his discipline and grade; it is important, therefore, to discover early on what these areas are since failure to perform well in them creates a poor impression.

Roles may be both formally and informally assigned (Ryle 1982). In the former case, one is likely to be told directly about them, and perhaps be given a handout delineating expectations and duties. But a wide range of informal roles may exist and the trainee should be on the alert for these. For instance, some may want him to be the Team Ignoramus and allow them to demonstrate their skill in educating him. Of course, informal roles such as this may conflict with other formal and informal expectations and requirements, in which case a certain delicacy of balance is required. In order that he may be alert to these aspects of his work, the incipient trainee should discuss his new job with his predecessor (in advance) and make a particular point of discovering what his wider functions could be.

Lack of experience in teamwork should be acknowledged without embarrassment. A statement that it does not seem easy (or even that it may seem unattractive) will probably be regarded as a hopeful first step by the team. Attempts to maintain a one-man unidisciplinary approach will certainly meet with formidable opposition and make life very uncomfortable for the whole team and especially for the individual concerned. It may also result in his patients getting a poor clinical deal, since the team will be inhibited or even prevented from offering what it may be good at; especially as, by and large, multidisciplinary teams are not heavily restrictive and may even allow a difficult individual too much leeway out of respect for his feelings. The appropriate level of humility probably comes hardest to doctors, who have usually been training longer than anybody else and may be getting a little tired of it after ten or fifteen years.

The Team's Experience

The opinion of one's predecessor about the job are useful not only in providing the kind of details described above, but also as a source of information about the predecessor himself. As the last occupant of the post he will have contributed to the team's experience of trainees and its mythology. Knowing something about what he was like may help to explain some odd reactions. For example, it need come as no surprise to the successor of someone who never wrote case summaries, if every team member stresses the importance of summaries in the first week.

A highly significant aspect of the team's expectations lies in the semi-mythical figure of the *Monster Trainee*, a composite of all the negative characteristics of one's discipline as seen by others and a number of specific negative characteristics of previous incumbents. It is worth discovering what the Monster Trainee's features are and making every effort to avoid manifesting them, since if some monster characteristics are identified by the team, the rest are likely to be ascribed as well. However, since many of the characteristics of the Monster will usually be discipline-appropriate behaviour occurring out of proportion, Monster status cannot be avoided by simply refusing to engage in potentially monstrous activities. Thus little credit will accrue to the doctor who claims ignorance of all forms of physical treatment in order to escape being stereotyped as overly concerned with matters organic. He may not become a Monster, but he will certainly be thought foolish. The team is looking for a balance which allows the proper exercise of individual expertise without implicit denial of the value and authority of other team members.

Working together

As Rowbottom & Hey (1978) point out, there are many approaches to teamwork, but it is worth trying to decide whether a particular team focuses on the use of shared skills (which Rowbottom & Hey call a unidisciplinary approach) or prefers to departmentalise functions. Another useful distinction to bear in mind is that between 'permanent teams', in which a relatively unchanging group regularly co-operates in assessment and casework, and 'networks' where the association is looser and particular groups are brought together for specific purposes. If the trainee and the team are to work well together, they need to learn the rules that each expects to be followed; for example, doctors may find that they do not simply decide who to admit and then tell the nurses, but that admissions are agreed by the team. Having identified the rules, each needs to conform itself somewhat to the other. The trainee probably has to do the greater part of the conforming, at least in the initial stages, since the team is larger and more powerful than he is and his supervisor is part of it. Even more importantly, this is actually part of the training experience and is necessary to facilitate learning.

The process of integration has many exciting aspects. It may release new potentials in the trainee which had previously been untapped or underused, enabling him to do some constructive and valuable work. Once he has established respect for himself amongst his colleagues, the trainee may even initiate ideas which will be of long-term benefit to the team. Here again a balance has to be sought between bland conformity to what any other team member wants at a particular moment and self-opinionation.

Supervision

All trainees will have a supervisor, who will be, in some sense, responsible for their work. A helpful supervisor will give the trainee a good start by letting him know what his special duties are and perhaps gently indicating areas of potential conflict. Regular (perhaps weekly) supervision meetings are crucial, since they can smooth integration and help the trainee to understand his supervisor and his supervisor's position in relation to the rest of the team. Since trainees are sometimes tarred with their supervisor's brush, it is as well to know what is in the tar! Trainees can use supervision both for clinical purposes and to discuss teamwork matters. The good supervisor will encourage discussion in both areas, since these are inextricably related.

Likewise, unit 'politics' should not be ignored and although others (and especially other trainees) will often prove more enlightening in this area, the supervisor may also be a good source of information. It is also worth noting the supervisor's view of when it is permissible (or even expected) to be in conflict or disagreement with members of other disciplines. Such disharmony may be viewed in a positive light, perhaps as a sign of character, whereas conflict in other contexts may be seen as trouble-making.

Difficulties arise if the supervisor is out of step with the team and actually expects non-team behaviour from his trainees. However, this situation will often be ameliorated by the support of other team members who recognise the difficult position of the trainee in such circumstances.

It is apposite at this point to mention the vexed question of leadership in multidisciplinary teams. All the professions involved in child mental health are 'asking for more involvement in decision taking, and to some extent in leadership' (Rhode 1984) while within the medical profession itself there is considerable debate as to the nature of medical responsibility in multidisciplinary teams (Rhode 1984). The, Mental Health Act (1983) has emphasised the central position of the consultant psychiatrist, at least in the compulsory treatment of mental disorder. So, for medical trainees at least, the non-autocratic style of many multidisciplinary team doctors may not be an appropriate role model for all settings. Certainly, there is a feeling among trainees preparing for the MRCPsych examination that they should give the impression of being 'in charge' of patient management, at least for the duration of the clinical exam. Trainees of other disciplines, who will ultimately practise in settings where medical staff are absent, may have precisely the opposite problem of finding that their training experience fails to provide sufficient practice in the independent formulation of management policy.

Observation

It is obvious that much training takes place through observing the 'experts' at work, followed by attempts at imitation, with the backing of direct supervision, independent reading and thought. In the same way, teamwork is probably best learnt by watching it in action and then trying things out. As a guide to thinking when observing team interactions it is worth bearing in mind the following questions:

Who wants what?
What techniques are being used to get it (for example, shouting, pulling rank, negotiation)?
Which members are in alliance?
Who is in opposition?
How is the alliance organised (for example, intradisciplinary links, personal friendship, etc)?
Did it work?

The active trainee will become involved in all sorts of negotiations and alliances to organise treatment programmes, admit patients, reorganise the tea rota or play particular games at the Christmas party. These are all learning experiences and it soon becomes clear that knowing the right answer is not enough – it has to be sold to the team.

Conclusion

Well-functioning multidisciplinary teams can provide a very stimulating and valuable training experience for junior staff of many disciplines. New lines of thought and development can be opened up and a wide range of experiences gained. As in any approach to psychiatric work, there are difficulties, losses and pitfalls, but a real willingness to overcome these and work with others in the interest of the patients results in the provision of a much broader and more rewarding experience than any one discipline could provide alone. Many would see the strengthening of multi-disciplinary approaches as providing the best means of improving mental health service provisions for those in need of them. Bettelheim, writing about the treatment team, comments 'When the goal of the common enterprise is to restore psychiatric patients to mental health, social solidarity is not just desirable and helpful, but a necessity'.

References and Further Reading

Ackerly B (1947) The clinic team. *American Journal of Orthopsychiatry*, **17**, 191–195

Bettelheim B (1974) *A Home for the Heart* London: Thames Hudson

Maudsley H (1902) *Life in Mind & Conduct.* London: Macmillan Co

Rhode P D (1984) The Future of the Consultant in Psychiatry - A continuing debate. *Bulletin of the Royal College of Psychiatrists*, **8**, 65–66

Rowbottom R & Hey A (1978) *Organisation of Services for the Mentally ill - a working paper.* Brunel Institute of Organisation & Social Studies

Ryle R (1982) Understanding Organisations. *Association for Child Psychology & Psychiatry News*, **11**, 1–5

Wells P (1984) Trainees in a Therapeutic Community for Adolescents. *Bulletin of the Royal College of Psychiatrists*, **8**, 67–69

World Health Organisation (1977) *Child Mental Health and Psychosocial Development. Report of a WHO Expert Committee.* World Health Organisation, Geneva

Wilson D N (1979) When is a team not a Team? *Apex. Journal of the British Institute for Mental Handicap*, **7**, 94

The Adolescent Unit
Edited by Derek Steinberg
© 1986 D. Steinberg

21 Developments in a Psychiatric Service for Adolescents

Derek Steinberg

Biographical note: Chapter 12

The diagram on page 210 (Figure 21.1) outlines how the clinical service at the Adolescent Unit at Bethlem works. It looks rather mechanical and impersonal, as flow charts do, but it represents what has emerged from several years of discussion and experiment, and is not an idealised blueprint. Each step says something about how we perceive our clientele and our relationships with them, and reflects a number of assumptions about adolescent problems and our response to them:-

1 Problems in adolescence are common (Graham & Rutter 1985; Parry-Jones 1985) but a specifically psychiatric response to them is often unnecessary (Steinberg 1981; 1982) and in particular admission to hospital is requested more often than it is needed (Steinberg *et al* 1981).

2 One of the relatively few indications for residential *psychiatric* care is complexity of the adolescent's problem, and moreover complexity that includes individual dysfunction (see Chapter 12, and Steinberg 1983).

3 Emergency admissions should be allowed for, but are rarely indicated, since the traditional hospital approach of a direct, rushed admission for close medical and nursing supervision is unnecessary for the majority of crises surrounding adolescents.

4 The reasons for admission have much to do with what is going on around the adolescent, and these factors need attention too, in order to help in ways that are appropriate. This approach has much in common with that developed by Bruggen and his colleagues (1973) and with methods based on crisis intervention (for example, Caplan 1961; Morrice 1976). However, we do not operate only on a social crisis or social systems model, but assume that the primary reason for a problem can also be disorder in the individual adolescent. Hence our assessment and management procedures allow for either possibility, or for both interacting.

5 Whatever the reason for admission, and however individual the disorder, every adolescent patient should have social, family and educational matters dealt with too, and these include (a) maintenance of the responsibilities, commitment, and skills of those already involved with the boy or girl, and his or her contact with them; (b) affirmation that the adolescent has a home address and never only a hospital

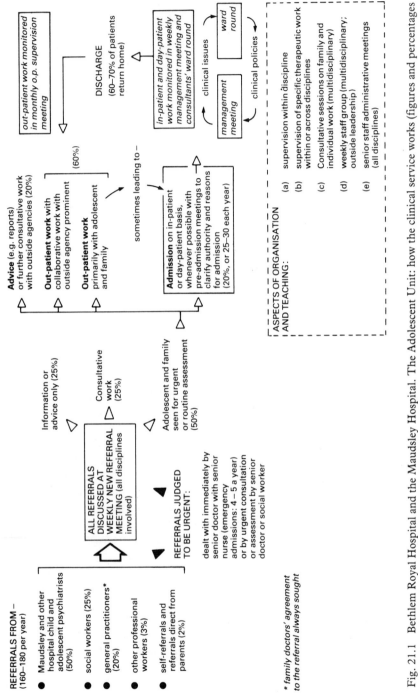

Fig. 21.1 Bethlem Royal Hospital and the Maudsley Hospital. The Adolescent Unit: how the clinical service works (figures and percentages are approximate: much variation from year to year)

address; (c) confirmation of authority to proceed with assessment, admission and treatment, whether this authority is the parents', the Social Service Department's, the adolescent's, or medical authority.

6 The response to the request for admission should have consultative (Caplan 1970; Dare *et al* 1982; Steinberg & Yule 1985) and diagnostic components (Steinberg 1983). That is to say, if at all possible and acceptable the referring agency and the adolescent unit team should engage in a joint appraisal of what those 'outside' should contribute, and what the unit should contribute. Further, this should continue throughout admission, in planning discharge and thereafter.

7 Within the adolescent unit there should similarly be a recognition of two distinct but complementary aspects of work: the treatment of individual disorder, on the one hand, and the maintenance of a milieu that enhances normal development on the other. In other words each adolescent has an individual treatment programme, and lives in a milieu which should be therapeutic and educational. Taking points 6 and 7 together, multidisciplinary work falls into three broad areas: individual diagnosis and treatment, if needed; milieu maintenance and development; and work with the people in the adolescent's life outside the unit.

Assessment

The multi-axial classification system forms a guide to our assessment procedure, although by no means accounts for the whole of it. In this system the boy or girl is assessed for the presence (or absence) of clinical disorder, and also in terms of specific developmental delay (for example, in reading), intellectual level, physical health and psychosocial circumstances. What we look for is evidence for individual problems or disorder in the adolescent, at any level, and features of the family and wider social setting which may have contributed and led to the referral. We assume that these latter family and social characteristics (for example, parental difficulties or a school's anxieties) may have contributed significantly to the process by which the boy or girl has become 'nominated' as a patient; and that responding to them is one aspect of reversing this process. Our assessment therefore includes a meeting between two of our staff and the family as a whole; followed by individual mental and physical state assessment of the adolescent. This dual approach operates on a sliding scale which is 'set' at the referral meeting. For some problems we will decide in advance that a whole family assessment would be the right approach, and individual assessment is reduced in scale or even, unusually, left out. For other types of referral (for example, concern about a young person's mental state) the individual assessment will predominate. This adaptability of our assessment procedure has not been developed without difficulty, for two reasons. Firstly, although 'individually-orientated' practitioners tend readily to see the point of both individual and family assessment, 'system-orientated' workers believe that by seeing the adolescent individually something important is thereby implied about child and family which can jeopardize their future family work.

The second difficulty concerns adaptability. There is no doubt that to adopt a strategy of flexibility, in which clinical judgement is used to decide how best to proceed in each child's case, can cause team anxiety and disputes. Provided that these are not allowed to become too time-consuming, my own view is that it is the interests of good practice and good teaching to discuss how best to approach assessment in each case, rather than adhere to a rigid routine.

A single-approach team, even if composed of members of different professions, is likely to be more comfortable with a standard approach to each new case, and indeed regard flexibility as a vice rather than a virtue. However, adaptability, practicality and recognition of the enormous differences between different people's cases are not only important characteristics of a genuinely multidisciplinary approach, but constitute its main *raison d'être*; it is a sound and well-founded way to respond to the diversity of people's problems, and needs to be asserted as such against the pressures of the more finely polished orthodoxies.

Our assessment leaves us with a view about the adolescent's psychiatric diagnosis, or lack of one; a list of problems in terms of disabilities and sources of concern, including further questions to answer; and a view of the family and other people involved – composed of their views and our views. Their views include not only what concerns them, and what they cannot do, but what they *can* do, and also their authority for us to proceed with our part of the work; for example, consent to admission and treatment. In effect we compile a 'job card'; work for us, work for the adolescent and work for the other involved adults, and this forms the basis for an agreement which is reviewed at intervals, along with progress made or not made. In principle this corresponds with the approach taken by many system-orientated units (for example, Bruggen *et al* 1973; Jones *et al* 1978). The difference, however, is that we allow within the family system for the systems within the individual, and regard this individual component as something about which the clinician can comment, and give advice.

Admission Policies and their Consequences

Over the years we have developed a policy of maximising the work done other than by admission. This includes recommending alternatives; offering consultation in the current crisis or in the longer term; encouraging other people's continuing work with the referred adolescent; and taking on as outpatients adolescents referred for admission. There are a number of important consequences of this way of working. The most obvious is that it is not always acceptable to the referring professional, who may feel let down when admission is not agreed, and reluctant to consider alternative strategies. This is a real dilemma, for individual professionals and for the planning of services. The referring professional worker will usually have already worked and thought hard about the alternatives to admission, and be understandably disinclined to allow also for the experience and opinions of those in the adolescent unit. It is true that the latter have not, at the moment of referral, met the boy or girl. However, they are likely to have experience of several hundred referrals each year, perhaps over many years. It is essential for an adolescent unit to be helpful, and equally essential for it to have an admissions policy which has integrity as well as being reasonably flexible. These two requirements are sometimes in conflict with each other, which is why, at this stage in the development of adolescent services, variation among units is valuable; we receive many referrals which 'are not worth referring to Dr X or unit Y'; but we know that Dr X and unit Y also take their turn at being the 'goodies' when referrers feel frustrated at the myth or the reality of our own unit. It is an understandable stage in the evolution of services for adolescents, but a disquieting one nonetheless; it is not one, in my own view, that will be properly met simply by establishing more 'beds'. (Steinberg, 1982).

Our approach to admissions raises a number of questions that have not been adequately researched, although we have studies in progress: firstly, what happens to young people referred for admission whom we do not admit? Secondly, what happens to young people referred for emergency admission, whether we admit them immediately or not? Thirdly, what are the benefits of inpatient treatment? Our impressions are that we certainly help a large proportion of those admitted, and although global follow-up studies are problematic we have been able to identify progress for individual groups (Bolton et al, 1983) while a study in progress shows that two-thirds of the young people we admit in fact return home (Turner et al, in preparation). As far as emergency admissions are concerned (defined as direct admissions within hours or days without prior planning) our very strong impression is that rather little is gained for a surprisingly large proportion; while quite a lot can be lost, including loss of the patient by premature discharge which might have been avoided by a planned approach.

An important consequence of the selective approach we operate is illustrated in Table 21.1. Our outpatient work is increasingly with young people with emotion and conduct problems (including school refusal, anorexia nervosa (Dare 1983) and overdoses) who would once have been more readily admitted; meanwhile, our inpatient and to some extent our daypatient population has tended to contain a larger number of more unwell young people, with a larger proportion having medication, being detained on sections of the Mental Health Act, having physical investigations, and suffering from psychotic disorders, than staff entering the field of adolescent psychiatry might have hoped to work with. This may be particularly true for non-psychiatrists. I would predict that most of the members of the Association for the Psychiatric Study of Adolescence, for example, would identify family therapy, or the therapeutic community, as the most useful and most acceptable options for work with the broad range of disturbed adolescents. However, I would also maintain that the clientele referred to in Table 1 represent a group of young people for whom a hospital setting, staffed by doctors and nurses, is most appropriate; and that a *primarily* family therapeutic or community-therapeutic facility does not need to be

Table 21.1   patients in the unit (February 1 1985)
(24 inpatient places plus 3-6 day places)

Individual diagnosis	Number of adolescents; age range 12–18 (m:f ratio in brackets)	Additional prominent problems
emotional and mixed disorders of emotions and conduct	5 (3:2)	2 with school refusal 2 with risk of self-injury
conduct disorder	3 (2:1)	1 with risk of self-injury
problem of personality development accompanying emotional disorder	3 (f)	
schizophrenic, schizo-affective or unspecified psychotic disorder	5 (3:2)	1 with serious risk of self-neglect* 2 with serious risk to others*
obsessional disorder	2 (f)	
anorexia nervosa	1 (f)	
transexual problem of personality development	1 (m)	with risk of self-injury

Additional data
(a) Three young people* detained on admission or later on a section of the Mental Health Act
(b) Seven on medication (5 neuroleptic; 1 antidepressant; 1 anticonvulsant)
(c) Six having specific physical health (as opposed to routine) investigations for cerebral disorder (4), renal function (1) and asthma (1)

based in a hospital, and does not need to be staffed by psychiatrists and psychiatric nurses.

Having said this, although we do not operate as a therapeutic community as ordinarily described (for example, see Rapoport 1960; Whiteley 1975; Clark 1977) our patients require management which gains from the experience of therapeutic communities, just as their management is also informed by the concepts and methods of family therapy. The unit has ward and community groups and a lively academic, creative and leisure programme run primarily by teachers, nurses and occupational therapists. The skills of the staff, and the 'mix' of the children, has to sustain an educational and therapeutic milieu suitable for bright and articulate children with emotional problems as well as adolescents who may be psychotic, brain damaged and inarticulate. Certainly we have found this mixture works in our small groups (Steinberg et al 1978). How far admission decisions may legitimately allow for what a relatively articulate youngster can *contribute* to the unit's atmosphere is an awkward ethical problem. Undoubtedly it would, and should, in a therapeutic community. The reverse is certainly true, however: there are times when the admission of one more aggressive or highly dependent young person cannot be safely managed by staff or the patient group, even when a 'bed' is technically available. Patients and their management programmes need staff time, not the simple availability of a mattress, as if in a Victorian field hospital. Nonetheless, ready bed availability and bed occupancy tend to be the crucial (if somewhat contradictory) standards by which hospital units are judged.

The general principle of minimising admissions extends also to shortening admissions. An outpatient and consultative service that helps avoid admission for all but a particularly difficult minority will also be able to return adolescents more speedily to their own home. Discharge policy as well as admission policy will therefore also affect the unit's patient population profoundly, with young people returning home as soon as they begin to improve and perhaps before they can become, for staff, more rewarding. Working with families in a way that shares what *we* can do and what *they* can do is likely to work in the same direction; indeed it should. This is no small matter, for staff recruitment, training and for fulfilment in work. A study is under way, led by Teresa Wilkinson and Derek Bolton and senior nursing colleagues, to explore what a community psychiatric nursing service can achieve in the way of shortening and avoiding admission to hospital; the impact on the unit of such changes is something we have already begun to look at.

Staff Training and Development

Another challenge for a treatment unit is achieving a reasonable balance between stability, and the security that goes with it, and change. Soon after beginning at the adolescent unit I began to lead a staff group (soon after taken by an outside consultant) whose brief was to look at and discuss developments and their impact on work and working relationships. It was expected that the unit would develop more family and consultative work, increase its teaching within the unit and outside (including the Course for Child and Adolescent Psychiatric Nursing), and increase its outpatient service. We also introduced small group work for all patients, began ward and community groups, and a more formal teaching, supervision and consultation structure for therapeutic work. We also mixed the two wards; they had previously been separate wards for boys and girls for some thirty years, and had developed differences of approach which went beyond sex difference alone. The former fact presented some difficulties, not the latter.

Throughout this period of change, partly contributing to it and partly resulting from it, the staff have changed too. The senior staff have been a relatively stable group, some seventeen people including several who have worked at the unit for around ten years or more, although senior nursing staff unfortunately tend to seek promotion after only two or three years. The great majority of the staff, however, are in training and stay for as little as 10-12 weeks (for example, psychology and nursing students) or six months (registrars). Social work students and senior registrars are attached for a year and around fifteen months respectively, while nursing assistants leave after a year or two. We therefore have to maintain stability and consistency in a setting where two thirds of the staff are in transit; there are arrivals and departures most weeks at a rate rather faster than the turnover of our patients.

Our staff group, administration and teaching programme therefore has this turnover to contend with. Another factor which challenges the integrity and cohesiveness of the unit is the allegiance of all staff to organisations and hierarchies other than the unit itself. The staff of the unit represent a coming together of the Maudsley and Bethlem Royal Hospitals; of the Children's and Adolescents' Department; of the Institute of Psychiatry; of the School of Nursing; of the local Department of Social Services, who employ our social workers; and of the Inner London Education Authority, which administers our school. In addition, fortunately, staff tend to be highly individualistic and properly ambitious people with academic and other commitments elsewhere. All this is stimulating, and to the good, but does not lead to stability or comfort. It also raises another question: multiplicity of purpose and an emphasis on teaching programmes and rotations are both desirable; indeed many non-teaching units aspire to this state, and the advantages for staff if not for patients are clear. However, at what point does this rate of turnover and fresh input reach a critical mass which begins to detract from the experience itself, and its value for training purposes?

My own role has two particular components: clinical responsibility for my patients, and a responsibility towards the unit as a therapeutic environment for patients and as a learning environment for staff. Both requirements need a balance between stability and set procedures, on the one hand, and questioning and exploration on the other.

There are a number of such factors in opposition to each other which have to be managed by an adolescent unit's leadership, and the outcome should be that of a dynamic equilibrium rather than a compromise. They include autocracy versus consensus in decision making; stasis and institutionalisation versus development; staff stability versus staff change; eclectic training and treatment versus the need to have a limited number of approaches, but undertaken with special skill; rigidity versus flexibility in procedures, and informality versus tight supervision and controls; following the rules versus individual imagination, judgement and flair; precision versus tolerance of ambiguity; a technological atmosphere versus a creative one. These are not listed as good and bad alternatives, but as antithetical tendencies out of which a good enough programme must be developed.

In the staff group, just as in individuals and teams working with adolescents, there is also a tendency to idealise or to denigrate: the unit is, for the moment, brilliant, or awful; a member of staff is wonderful, or dreadful; our work is successful, or a failure; this or that outside office or department is 'good' or 'bad'. It is important that there are a sufficient number of mature staff to handle such feelings, which can become very powerful, and which are connected with the ambivalent and alternating projected feelings that have their origins in adolescent disturbance: feeling ill becomes mirrored as ill feeling, and rational judgements become difficult. These and many other feelings are for the staff group to address.

Soon after starting the group we asked John Foskett to lead it as an outside consultant (Chapter 17), and we began a separate administrative meeting to deal with policies and planning. This meeting has an agenda and minutes; the staff group ends without decisions, except for the conclusions that individuals make for themselves, in which sense the group is essentially consultative (Steinberg & Yule 1985). For several years we had a similar group for senior staff, which dealt with senior staff working relationships and respective roles, the supervision of junior staff and longer term issues which we wanted to separate from discussion with more transient staff members. Once or twice a year we hold staff training days, taken by outside consultants, and using group experiential techniques to examine such topics as communication, professional roles, sex differences and decision making. It would be desirable but difficult to evaluate all these group activities; however, I have no doubt about their value at least for teaching staff about the realities of social and inter-professional relationships in treatment organisations, particularly where more than one profession and several grades of seniority are involved.

Teaching also takes place in individual supervision (sometimes across disciplines), in seminars and conferences and in direct supervision of family work and social skills training using personal report, audiovisual methods and the one-way screen. We have also introduced consultative meetings for family therapy and individual psychotherapy (described by Christopher Dare in chapter 9 and Peter Wilson in chapter 10, respectively). Staff are encouraged to attend outside courses and conferences as well as teaching elsewhere in the hospital. We are in the fortunate position of having the expectation that teaching will be an important priority for the unit. Certainly, our 'production' includes some 60 or so professional workers each year undergoing advanced training in the various disciplines, a figure which compares with the number of inpatients and daypatients discharged. Nevertheless, the practicalities of making time for teaching put it into competition with finding time for research and clinical work. Nurses in particular are vulnerable to the assumption that 'service' needs come first. It is perhaps easy to say that the clinical service must have priority; it is equally easy to make the point that without teaching and research clinical work ceases to be feasible. In fact the three are totally interdependent, and a unit or team programme which skimps on one drains the value of all three.

Making time for systematic research has its difficulties, not least because of the sustained effort and attention to detail needed. Interruptions to deal with clinical emergencies or telephone calls will make a nominal 'research afternoon' meaningless, and attention must be paid to making sure that staff able and willing to undertake research have the time and space in which to do it. Certainly this is an area in which, I feel, our own service should improve. Not everyone has the aptitude or inclination for large-scale enquiries, but curiosity about our clientele and our methods should be intrinsic to our work, which gains in every way from being conducted in a spirit of imaginative enquiry. It is a truism, and true, that every patient and every intervention is unique, and therefore an experiment. Even the simple but useful technique of defining problems, setting goals and monitoring their achievement is a beginning to systematic study, and can be applied to everything we do, even psychodynamic work.

Time, Space, and Staff Support

Imaginative timetabling is unusual. Department and unit programmes tend to grow in ramshackle, chaotic patterns, with more and more 'absolutely vital' sessions being crammed in until there is no room for any more. Spaces in other people's timetables, left for seeing patients, talking to colleagues, or lunch, can be eyed with curiosity and a little envy by people whose own programmes have got out of hand. Senior staff have a responsibility to ensure that the intelligent planning of timetables replaces the obsessional or frenetic 'squeezing in' of one more service commitment or one more teaching session or course. The need for comprehensive training, or comprehensive service, must be balanced against the need to undertake both properly, which takes time. I do not believe that a day which is composed of dashing from meeting to meeting to fulfil everybody's expectations is in anybody's interests. It certainly does not help patients, and can undermine interest and curiosity rather than stimulate them. It sometimes seems a way of avoiding real work, clinical or academic, despite an impression of busyness. Cherished gatherings, therefore, to which multidisciplinary work is particularly vulnerable, may have to be dropped or made less frequent to make room for new activities which really represent developments in teaching or practice. Of course it is difficult, but the point I am making is that there should be a sense of responsibility among senior people for imaginative timetabling as a positive contribution to teaching and work, rather than regarding the timetable problem as the irritating intrusion of reality.

'Staff support' is an elusive feature of organisations. Organising time, space and the material needs of staff (including furnishing and decoration and proper technical aids for administrative work) is I believe as important as dealing with staff group dynamics. Personal timetabling and professional self-management in general should be a component of supervision within disciplines. My experience of colleagues in this broad field is that they tend to be self-motivated and conscientious rather than the reverse, and need to be taught how to say 'no', and how to make time for themselves. Again, this is in patients' interests, not least because even the most disillusioned adolescent takes courage from being with adults who enjoy their work, and can look after themselves.

Multidisciplinary Work or Teamwork?

It should not be assumed that *work* equals *teamwork* in multidisciplinary settings. Indeed, the value of having a number of people with quite different perspectives and backgrounds working together may be substantially reduced if there is an explicit or implicit drive to operate primarily as a team.

'Team' has its origins in the Old English term for a set of draught animals yoked together, and presumably at their most effective when moving the same load in the same direction. One should not make too much of early etymology; nonetheless, the notion of the team as unified in a common purpose is still with us, with comforting intimations of democracy and mutual co-operation too. The *team* must work coherently, with a high level of internal and external consistency, and it achieves this if its members more or less think alike, with genuine disagreement regarded as a puzzling or unwelcome distraction; or by accepting direction from an authoritative leadership. Of course there will be discussion, and often its members will be drawn from different disciplines, but there will be no serious intellectual challenge to the team's basic assumptions.

The *multidisciplinary working group*, if it takes its diversity seriously, is eclectic, adaptable, untidy and makes room for real argument as opposed to ideological hair-splitting. It is not without its own ideology, taking for granted that human life and development is complex, wayward and individualistic and that professional responses have therefore to be adaptable. Its strength is in generating ideas and methods: teaching and research. To get organised, and carry out tasks, the multidisciplinary working group needs sub-groups working as teams. Some are 'standing teams', such as the nursing team, the teaching team, or various administrative groups; some are *ad hoc*, for example, those groups of three or four people recruited from the wider group to undertake a programme of treatment with a patient and family.

There is a need for both team (uniformity) and multidisciplinary working group (diversity) methods in a healthy organisation which is both innovative and effective. Therapeutic communities and single-approach units will tend towards the former, and eclectic units will tend towards the latter, 'budding off' teams for specific purposes. In this respect it needs to be said that milieu-maintenance in any setting is a team-type function.

Developments

Improvements in school-based and home-based help for adolescents, including better training and status for 'front-line' staff, will affect the number of inpatient places that will be needed. I believe the overall number will probably diminish, with some re-distribution of available places to provide more accessible services; and in the long run I cannot see *hospital-based* units being justified unless they provide a primarily general psychiatric service. Of the young people who cannot be managed at home, the great majority would be better provided for by socially-based 'crisis' and assessment units, therapeutic communities, schools, children's homes and hostels, which would work in liaison with each other, and preferably close to the communities they serve.

The general psychiatric adolescent unit is likely to be an exciting and absorbing as well as demanding place, with endless temptations for looking inwards rather than outwards. This should be resisted, and these units should do their best to develop in a dual way, on the one hand maintaining the setting as one which is stimulating and innovative and encourages staff and patient development; on the other helping staff, patients (and potential patients) to function away from the institution. For reasons which are referred to many times in this book, this is easier said than done.

Multidisciplinary work has about it the feel of professional groups in transition. In the short term, units that employ many disciplines should consider their management structure, and which professions should be central, which more peripheral and which available on a visiting, liaison and consultative basis; this move would free staff and energy for more practice based away from the unit. If the choice is between centralised, complex organisations and many smaller, simpler units closer to the community, my own recommendation would be for the latter. In the long term, the drift towards ever-finer divisions and sub-divisions into specialisation should surely be reversed, so that through the experience of the period of super-specialisation we can encourage better-trained generalists.

The single most important quality of units, services and staff should be the capacity for new learning and change; the sort of thing we expect of our clientele. Innovative experiments in institutions should be positively encouraged, even rewarded, and the threat of loss of resources during experimental transition (for example, from 'beds' to community based work) removed or at least put on a predictable basis. The results of large-scale planning have not been generally impressive. Smaller, more autonomous developments, with evaluation built in, are worth trying; in structure they could usefully learn from those children's building games which can quite easily connect up with and detach from each other. This could well be a better way to build networks up from the roots, rather than from some grand design. Within such developments, the most valuable contribution of the larger, more centralised multidisciplinary service would be not so much a wonderful opportunity to involve everyone in everything with everyone in charge, but to learn and to teach.

References and Further Reading

Barker P (ed) (1974) *The Residential Psychiatric Treatment of Children*. London, Crosby Lockwood/Staples

Bolton D, Collins S & Steinberg D (1983) The treatment of obsessive-compulsive disorder in adolescence: a report of 15 cases. *British Journal of Psychiatry*, **142**, 456-464

Bruggen P, Byng-Hall J & Pitt-Aikens T (1973) The reason for admission as a focus of work in an adolescent unit. *British Journal of Psychiatry*, **122**, 319-329

Caplan G (1961) *An Approach to Community Mental Health*. London: Tavistock Publications

Caplan G (1970) *The Theory and Practice of Mental Health Consultation*. London: Tavistock Publications

Clark D H (1977) The therapeutic community. *British Journal of Psychiatry*, **13**, 553-564

Dare C (1983) Family therapy for families containing an anorectic youngster. In *Understanding Anorexia Nervosa and Bulimia. The 4th Ross Conference on Medical Research*. Ohio: Ross Laboratories

Dare C (1985) Family therapy. In M Rutter & L Hersov (eds) *Child and Adolescent Psychiatry: Modern Approaches*. Oxford: Blackwell, pp 809-825

Dare C, Ryle R, Steinberg D & Yule W (eds) (1982) Consultation from child and adolescent psychiatric settings. *News of the Association for Child Psychology and Psychiatry*, No 11

Graham P & Rutter M (1985) Adolescent disorders. In M Rutter & L Hersov (eds) *Child and Adolescent Psychiatry: Modern Approaches*. Oxford: Blackwell, pp 317-367

Hersov L & Bentovim A (1985) Inpatient and day-hospital units. In M Rutter & L Hersov (eds) *Child and Adolescent Psychiatry: Modern Approaches*. Oxford: Blackwell, pp 766-779

Heacock D R (ed) (1980) *A Psychodynamic Approach to Adolescent Psychiatry: the Mount Sinai Experience*. New York: Marcel Dekker

Jones R M, Allen D J, Wells P G & Morris A (1978) An adolescent unit assessed: attitudes to a treatment experience for adolescents and their families. *Journal of Adolescence*, **1**(4), 371-383

Kreeger L (ed) (1975) *The Large Group: Dynamics and Therapy*. London: Constable

Martin D V (1962) *Adventure in Psychiatry. Social Change in a Mental Hospital.* Oxford: Cassirer

Morrice J K W (1976) *Crisis Intervention: Studies in Community Care*. Oxford: Pergamon

Parry-Jones W L (1985) Adolescent disturbance. In M Rutter & L Hersov (eds) *Child and Adolescent Psychiatry: Modern Approaches*. Oxford: Blackwell, pp 584-598

Rapoport R N (1960). *Community as Doctor*. London: Tavistock

Rutter M (1979) *Changing Youth in a Changing Society. Patterns of Adolescent Development and Disorder*. London: Nuffield Provincial Hospitals Trust

Steinberg D (1981) *Using Child Psychiatry: the Functions and Operations of a Specialty*. London: Hodder & Stoughton

Steinberg D (1982) Treatment, training, care or control? The functions of adolescent units. *British Journal of Psychiatry*, **141**, 306-309

Steinberg D (1983) *The Clinical Psychiatry of Adolescence. Clinical Work from a Social and Developmental Perspective*. Chichester: Wiley

Steinberg D & Yule W (1985) Consultative work. In M Rutter & L Hersov (eds) *Child and Adolescent Psychiatry: Modern Approaches*. Oxford: Blackwell, pp 914-926

Steinberg D, Galhenage D P C & Robinson S C (1981) Two years' referrals to a regional adolescent unit: some implications for psychiatric services. *Social Science & Medicinc*, **15**, 113-122

Steinberg D, Merry J & Collins S (1978) The introduction of small group work to an adolescent unit. *Journal of Adolescence*, **1**, 331-344

Turner T H, Dossetter D, Bates R (In preparation). The early outcome of adolescent admission - a report of 100 cases.

Whiteley J S (1975) The large group as a medium for sociotherapy. In L Kreeger (ed) *The Large Group*. London: Constable

Author Index

223

Subject Index

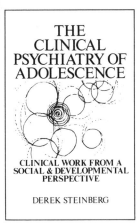

THE
CLINICAL
PSYCHIATRY OF
ADOLESCENCE

CLINICAL WORK FROM A
SOCIAL & DEVELOPMENTAL
PERSPECTIVE

DEREK STEINBERG

THE CLINICAL PSYCHIATRY OF ADOLESCENCE

Clinical Work from a Social and Developmental Perspective

by **D. Steinberg,**
Consultant Psychiatrist, Adolescent Unit, Bethlem Royal Hospital and the Maudsley Hospital, London

Disturbed adolescents present a very wide range of problems and many different sorts of service and professional worker are available to help them. The main focus of this book is the special contribution of clinical psychiatry to the care of some adolescents, and the ways in which clinical psychiatrists can collaborate with other workers with young people. The book therefore takes a broad perspective, describing the principles and practice of clinical work with young people in the context of their other needs. To this end the book discusses not only clinical diagnosis and a wide range of methods of psychiatric treatment, but also the range of other services for young people and the history of their growth, and a number of theories of physical, social, intellectual and emotional development.
(Wiley Series on Studies in Child Psychiatry)

Contents:
Preface: Guide to the Book; PART I: DIAGNOSIS: Concepts of Disorder and the Presentation of Problems; Adolescent Psychiatry in Perspective; Clinical Psychiatry in Relation to the Problems of Adolescence; The Emergence of Problems I: Development; The Emergence of Problems II: The Referral Process; A System for Assessment; The Diagnostic Formulation; PART II: PROBLEMS: Categories of Problem; Categories of Disorder; Problems of Feeling and Behaviour; Anorexia Nervosa, Obesity, and Other Disorders of Eating; Enuresis, Encopresis and Tics; Depressive Disorders; Affective and Schizophrenic Psychoses and Major Disorders of Personality Development; Autism, Mental Retardation and Learning Disabilities; Physical Problems; PART III: MANAGEMENT: Strategies of Intervention; Psychodynamic, Social, and Behavioural Approaches; Aspects of Residential Treatment; Medication and Other Physical Treatments; Consultation, Collaboration, Teaching and Learning; References; Index.

'. . . a scholarly work with a comprehensive list of references written by one of the leading teachers in the field. It should find a place in libraries of all departments of psychiatry and of all adolescent psychiatry units.'

The Lancet

0 471 10314 4   412pp   1983